The OA Relief Diet

Simple Foods, Snacks, Supplements, and Smart Eating Out Choices to Reduce Joint Pain Naturally

By
LEON EDWARD

Copyright © 2025 Leon Edward. All rights reserved.

ISBN ebook: 979-8-9925482-0-4
ISBN paperback: 979-8-9925482-1-1

No part of this book may be copied, reproduced, stored, or transmitted in any form—electronic, mechanical, photocopying, recording, or otherwise—without the author's prior written permission, except for brief excerpts used in reviews or educational references.

While every effort has been made to ensure the accuracy of this book at the time of publication, the author and publisher assume no responsibility for errors, omissions, or changes in medical or dietary guidelines after publication.

This book provides general information on the subject matter and is not intended as medical or dietary advice. The publisher is not engaged in rendering professional or medical services. Readers should consult a qualified health professional for personalized advice.

References to websites, organizations, or external resources are provided for informational purposes only and do not imply endorsement or affiliation. The author and publisher are not responsible for content changes, broken links, or discontinued services.

The OA Relief Diet

Simple Foods, Snacks, Supplements, and Smart Eating Out Choices to Reduce Joint Pain Naturally

Table of Contents

Introduction 1
   Brief overview of OA and diet's role in joint health 1
   What to expect from this book 3

Chapter 1: Understanding Osteoarthritis & Joint Pain 7
   The Science Behind OA (cartilage breakdown,
   inflammation, joint degeneration) 7
   Common Symptoms & Impact on Daily Life
   (stiffness, pain, mobility challenges) 10

Chapter 2: How Diet Affects OA & Inflammation 13
   The Link Between Food & Joint Health
   (chronic inflammation & pain) 13
   Key Nutrients for OA Relief
   (omega-3s, antioxidants, collagen-building foods) 16

Chapter 3: Anti-Inflammatory Foods for OA 19
   Best Fruits & Vegetables for Joint Health 19
   Whole Grains & Lean Proteins That Reduce Inflammation 21

Chapter 4: Easy, No-Cook Snacks for OA Support 25
   Snack Ideas Rich in Omega-3s & Joint-Healthy Nutrients 25
   Building a Balanced OA-Friendly Snack Box 27

Chapter 5: The Power of Hydration & Joint Lubrication 31
   Why Water is Essential for Cartilage Health 31
   Hydrating Beverages & Their Benefits (bone broth, herbal teas, etc.) 34

Chapter 6: Key Supplements for OA Relief 37
   Turmeric & Black Pepper: A Natural Anti-Inflammatory 37
   Omega-3 Fatty Acids, Vitamin D, and Glucosamine for Joint Health 40
   Avocado-Soybean Unsaponifiables (ASU) &
   Their Role in Cartilage Protection 42

Chapter 7: Budget-Friendly Grocery Shopping for
OA-Friendly Eating 46
    Smart Shopping Strategies (finding discounts,
    bulk buying, frozen alternatives) 46
    Best Affordable OA-Friendly Foods 49

Chapter 8: Eating Out with OA – Smart Restaurant &
Fast Food Choices 52
    How to Identify OA-Friendly Restaurant Dishes 52
    Navigating Menus & Making Healthier Choices on a Budget 55
    Good vs. Bad Restaurant Food Cheat Sheet 57

Chapter 9: Incorporating Dietary Changes Without Meal Prep 60
    Simple Swaps for an Anti-Inflammatory Diet 60
    Practical Eating Tips for Busy Lifestyles 62

Chapter 10: Sustainable Dietary Habits for Long-Term OA Relief 66
    Building a Balanced OA Diet Without Stress 66
    Maintaining Motivation & Making Small, Lasting Changes 69

Chapter 11: Real-Life Success Stories & Testimonials 73
    Stories from OA Patients Who Improved Joint Health
    Through Diet 73
    Lessons Learned & Encouraging Takeaways 76

Chapter 12: Frequently Asked Questions About Diet & OA 79
    Common Concerns About OA, Inflammation & Food 79
    Expert Answers & Clarifications 82

Conclusion 85
    Key Takeaways & Final Encouragement 85

Appendix A: Resources & Further Reading 87
    Recommended Books, Websites, and Research Papers 87
    Online support groups for OA-friendly diet & lifestyle 90
    From the Author 92

References 95

Introduction

Osteoarthritis (OA) is a common joint condition that affects many adults, particularly those over 50, leading to discomfort, inflammation, and reduced mobility. It can make everyday tasks challenging, but there's good news: diet can play a significant role in managing these symptoms. This book aims to be your practical guide to naturally reducing joint pain and inflammation, focusing on easy dietary changes that won't overwhelm you with complex meal preparations. Whether you're a caregiver, a senior on a budget, or simply looking to enhance your joint health through nutrition, you'll find valuable insights into the powerful effects of anti-inflammatory foods, supplements, and smart choices when dining out. Our goal is to empower you with sustainable strategies that fit your lifestyle, helping you make gradual changes towards improved joint health and a better quality of life. By understanding the connection between what you eat and how your joints feel, you'll be better equipped to support your body's natural healing processes through everyday food choices.

Brief overview of OA and diet's role in joint health

Osteoarthritis (OA) is the most common form of arthritis, affecting millions worldwide, especially those over the age of 50 (Hunter & Bierma-Zeinstra, 2019). It represents a significant challenge in daily life for many, characterized by pain, stiffness, and reduced mobility due to the breakdown of cartilage in joints. While there's no cure for OA, managing symptoms and improving quality of life is possible through a holistic approach which includes diet as a key component. This book aims to shed light on how dietary choices can play a pivotal role in managing OA symptoms.

Diet isn't just about sustenance, it's about fueling your body with the right nutrients to promote overall health. For OA patients, the connection between what you eat and how your joints feel is particularly significant. Chronic inflammation, a hallmark of OA, can be exacerbated or alleviated by certain foods. This opens a pathway for dietary adjustments as a natural way to manage pain and inflammation (Zhang et al., 2018).

Adopting an anti-inflammatory diet can help cushion the impact of OA. Research suggests that certain nutrients, such as omega-3 fatty acids, antioxidants, and collagen-building foods can reduce inflammation and promote joint health (Messier et al., 2019). Omega-3s, found in fatty fish like salmon, help combat inflammation at a cellular level. Similarly, antioxidants found in fruits and vegetables help neutralize free radicals, which are known to contribute to inflammation and degenerative diseases.

On the other hand, some foods can exacerbate joint pain and inflammation. Excessive consumption of processed foods, high in sugars and unhealthy fats, are known to trigger inflammatory responses in the body (Zhang et al., 2018). Here, the role of a carefully considered diet comes into play, making it critical to understand which foods to embrace and which to avoid.

A mindful approach to eating doesn't have to be complex or time-consuming. For seniors, and particularly for those managing OA, it's important to integrate dietary changes in a way that's sustainable and easy to follow. Simple swaps, like choosing whole grains over refined carbohydrates, can significantly contribute to inflammation reduction, making daily meals healthier without adding complexity to preparation.

The upcoming chapters in this book delve into various dietary strategies that support joint health. From snack ideas rich in omega-3s to navigating restaurant menus, these strategies aim to empower you with the knowledge to make changes that suit your lifestyle. And for caregivers and family members, understanding these dietary principles can play a vital role in supporting loved ones dealing with OA.

Ensuring proper hydration is another crucial element that often goes unnoticed but can significantly affect joint function and lubrication. Staying hydrated aids in maintaining the viscosity of synovial fluid, which is essential for cushioning the joints. Integrating hydration habits along with dietary changes can optimize joint health and improve mobility.

All these elements come together to form a comprehensive dietary approach to managing osteoarthritis. The goal is not just to offer temporary relief but to facilitate long-lasting dietary habits that promote a natural reduction in OA symptoms. Through thoughtful food choices and by understanding your body's nutritional needs, you can manage joint health in a more manageable and natural way.

This structured guide aims to walk alongside you in your OA management journey, providing practical advice and insights drawn from scientific evidence and real-life success stories. This combination of empathetic support and scientific grounding aims to motivate and inspire positive change, showing that managing OA naturally through diet is truly within reach.

What to expect from this book

Embarking on the journey to manage osteoarthritis (OA) naturally through diet and lifestyle modifications is an empowering step. Our book serves as a comprehensive guide, providing you with actionable insights and practical strategies designed specifically for adults 50 and over, their caregivers, budget-conscious seniors, and those looking for simple and natural dietary solutions. This section of the introduction will set the stage for what you'll gain from the pages that follow.

First and foremost, expect to deepen your understanding of osteoarthritis and joint pain. We'll explore the science behind OA, presenting information in an accessible way that helps make sense of the mechanics of joint degeneration, cartilage breakdown, and inflammation. Grasping these fundamentals is essential, as it lays the framework for how dietary choices can profoundly influence joint health. By understanding the role that inflammation plays in OA, you can better appreciate how diet impacts your day-to-day mobility and comfort.

As you continue through the chapters, you'll find in-depth discussions on how diet and nutrition affect OA and inflammation. We'll uncover the intrinsic link between what you eat and how your joints feel, guided by scientific evidence. You'll learn about the specific nutrients that can aid in reducing joint pain, such as omega-3 fatty acids and powerful antioxidants. This knowledge is not presented simply as a set of facts but as a toolkit to empower you to make informed decisions that can lead to meaningful improvements in joint health.

Beyond the theoretical, our book is packed with practical, hands-on advice. Expect to discover a plethora of anti-inflammatory foods that can become staples in your diet. We'll guide you on choosing the right fruits, vegetables, whole grains, and proteins that actively work to reduce inflammation. The emphasis is on simplicity and accessibility, ensuring that the transition to a joint-healthy diet feels attainable rather than overwhelming.

For those who may not have the time or inclination to spend hours in the kitchen, we've included easy, no-cook snack ideas. These are snack options that are not only rich in essential nutrients but also easy to prepare. Whether you want to build an anti-inflammatory snack box or need quick ideas for those busy days, we've got you covered.

We also delve into the critical, yet often overlooked, role of hydration. Expect to learn why staying hydrated is crucial for maintaining cartilage health and joint lubrication. We'll explore a variety of hydrating beverages—from simple water to more flavorful options like bone broth and herbal teas—that can fit seamlessly into your daily routine.

The book will also equip you with knowledge about beneficial supplements. Not just any supplements, but those that are backed by research for their efficacy in providing OA relief. We'll cover familiar names like turmeric, omega-3 fatty acids, and glucosamine, and also introduce you to options like Avocado-Soybean Unsaponifiables (ASU), explaining how these can play a part in protecting cartilage and reducing inflammation.

Considering budget-friendly options is one of our core goals. You can expect a dedicated chapter on smart grocery shopping strategies for purchasing OA-friendly foods without breaking the bank. Tips on finding discounts, buying in bulk, and selecting frozen alternatives can help you eat well while staying within budget. Our aim is to make sure financial constraints don't become a barrier to healthier eating.

For moments when cooking isn't an option, we'll guide you on how to eat out without derailing your joint health goals. Learn to navigate restaurant menus with confidence, identifying dishes that align with your dietary needs and recognizing which meals to avoid. This chapter offers practical advice for making informed choices, even when you're on the go.

Incorporating dietary changes without intensive meal prep is made simpler through a chapter dedicated to quick swaps and practical tips. This section will empower you with ways to adapt your diet seamlessly into a busy lifestyle, suggesting straightforward adjustments that don't require a significant overhaul of your current eating habits.

One of the book's core promises is sustainability. We discuss how to build lasting dietary habits that can provide long-term relief from OA. By setting small, achievable goals, you can maintain motivation and see continuous improvement in joint health over time. This is not a temporary fix but a path toward sustained well-being.

Finally, be inspired by real-life success stories and testimonials from individuals who have transformed their joint health through diet changes. These stories serve as a reminder that you're not alone on this journey and demonstrate the tangible benefits that dietary modifications can bring.

Overall, expect this book to be a trusted companion in your quest for natural joint pain relief. It's structured not only to provide scientific and dietary guidance but also to offer empathy and understanding. You have the power to take control of your joint health, and this book aims to provide the tools and inspiration to do just that.

Chapter 1:
Understanding Osteoarthritis & Joint Pain

Osteoarthritis (OA) is a complex condition characterized by the breakdown of joint cartilage and the accompanying inflammation and pain that often result from this degeneration (Felson et al., 2000). As the most common form of arthritis, OA significantly impacts the daily lives of those over 50, causing symptoms like stiffness, persistent pain, and reduced mobility. These symptoms can interfere with simple activities, from walking to opening jars. Understanding the science behind OA reveals that it's not just the wear and tear but also biochemical changes in the joint that drive this condition (Hunter & Bierma-Zeinstra, 2019). This chapter explores these underlying mechanisms to provide a foundation for managing joint pain naturally. Integrating an understanding of cartilage breakdown and joint degeneration with practical dietary solutions is key to reducing inflammation and enhancing joint health, offering a path toward improved quality of life.

The Science Behind OA (cartilage breakdown, inflammation, joint degeneration)

Understanding osteoarthritis (OA) is vital for anyone looking to manage joint pain, especially through dietary changes. Let's dive into the science behind OA, focusing specifically on cartilage breakdown, inflammation, and joint degeneration.

Cartilage serves as the cushion in our joints, facilitating smooth movement and absorbing stress when you move. Over time, due to aging, wear and tear, or injury, this cartilage begins to wear down, leading to OA. In simple terms, imagine the cartilage as a shock absorber in a car. When it's new, it provides a seamless ride, but as it wears out, every bump becomes more pronounced, much like the discomfort one feels as cartilage breaks down. The thinning of this cartilage not only reduces joint functionality but also triggers pain as bones start to rub against each other (Brandt et al., 2009).

Inflammation is another significant player in the progression of OA. Normally, inflammation is the body's response to injury or infection, but in the case of OA, it becomes a chronic condition. This ongoing inflammation contributes to more rapid cartilage degradation. The process involves immune cells that release cytokines and enzymes, further eroding the cartilage and surrounding structures (Felson, 2004). Picture it like a small fire that, when left unchecked, starts consuming everything around it.

Joint degeneration isn't limited to the loss of cartilage alone. As the disease progresses, the bones undergo changes too. The exposed bone surfaces can develop osteophytes, which are small, bony growths that add to the stiffness and pain. Furthermore, the joint lining becomes inflamed, and the synovial fluid, essential for lubrication, may decrease or become less effective. This series of changes impedes the joint's ability to function normally, causing pain and limiting mobility (Felson, 2004). It's an intricate process where every component of the joint starts interacting in ways they were never meant to.

OA isn't uniform; it doesn't present the same way in everyone. Factors such as genetics, body weight, and previous injuries can influence both the onset and severity of the disease. For instance, obesity is a well-recognized risk factor, not only because of the added mechanical stress on the joints but also due to the pro-inflammatory substances secreted by adipose tissue (Messier et al., 2005). Weight management, therefore, plays a crucial role in mitigating the effects of OA.

Given this complex interplay of factors, interventions need to be multifaceted. While traditional treatments often focus on pain relief and anti-inflammatory medications, there's growing interest in how lifestyle, particularly diet, can influence the disease process. Certain nutrients have been shown to support cartilage health and reduce inflammation, potentially slowing the progression of OA. For example, Omega-3 fatty acids are known for their anti-inflammatory properties and may help in reducing the pain and inflammation associated with OA. Similarly, antioxidants present in fruits and vegetables can protect joint tissues from oxidative stress and further damage (Messier et al., 2005).

An interesting area of research is the impact of diet on the gut microbiome and its indirect effect on inflammation and joint health. A diet high in fiber, rich in fruits, vegetables, and whole grains, supports a healthy gut microbiome, which in turn can modulate inflammatory responses throughout the body. It's a holistic approach, understanding that what you eat not only affects your digestive health but also your joints (Felson, 2004).

Moreover, supplements like glucosamine and chondroitin, which are natural compounds found in cartilage, have been studied for their potential to enhance joint health and alleviate symptoms. Although evidence on their efficacy varies, many people with OA use them, hoping to support their joint's structural integrity (Brandt et al., 2009).

The science behind OA reveals a complex disease that requires a comprehensive strategy to manage effectively. By focusing on the mechanisms of cartilage breakdown and inflammation, individuals can make informed choices about their diet and lifestyle. Incorporating anti-inflammatory foods, maintaining a healthy weight, and possibly using supplements under medical guidance can make a tangible difference in managing OA. It's all about understanding these processes and being proactive in addressing them. While OA is a common issue, particularly as we age, staying informed empowers you to take control and navigate your journey towards better joint health.

Common Symptoms & Impact on Daily Life (stiffness, pain, mobility challenges)

Osteoarthritis (OA) can manifest through a range of symptoms that not only vary in intensity but also significantly affect daily life. At the core of these symptoms are stiffness, pain, and mobility challenges, which together paint a picture of the lived experience of someone with OA. Understanding these symptoms is crucial for devising effective management strategies and fostering empathy among caregivers and families.

Stiffness is often one of the first noticeable symptoms of osteoarthritis. Many individuals find that it is most pronounced in the morning or after periods of inactivity. This stiffness results from the lack of joint lubrication, a consequence of the degeneration of cartilage—something that is exacerbated by the inflammatory processes at play in OA (Felson, 2006). While stiffness can ease as the day progresses, it can be particularly debilitating, affecting the ability to perform simple activities like getting out of bed or standing up from a chair.

Pain is arguably the most distressing symptom for those with osteoarthritis. It arises not just from inflammation but also from the mechanical wear and tear on the joint surfaces. Pain can be sharp or dull and may vary throughout the day depending on activity levels. For some, it is a constant companion, but for others, it comes and goes. Regardless of its pattern, pain makes activities that were once done with ease—such as climbing stairs or walking—challenging and often induces a cycle of inactivity exacerbating stiffness and muscle weakness (Hochberg et al., 1995).

The impact of pain on daily life cannot be overstated. It's more than just a physical experience; it has emotional and psychological repercussions. Chronic pain often leads to frustration and can contribute to mood disorders, including depression and anxiety. These emotional burdens add another layer of complexity to managing osteoarthritis, highlighting the importance of a holistic approach that addresses both the physical and mental aspects of the condition.

Mobility challenges are a direct consequence of both pain and stiffness. As cartilage deteriorates, the friction between bones increases, making joint movement awkward and sometimes unbearable. Mobility challenges can lead to a sedentary lifestyle, reducing overall fitness and leading to weight gain, which further aggravates joint pain and increases the burden on affected joints. This vicious cycle of inactivity, pain, and weight gain necessitates targeted interventions to break the pattern (Hunter & Bierma-Zeinstra, 2019).

Beyond these immediate physical symptoms, osteoarthritis affects various aspects of daily living. For instance, tasks that require fine motor skills, such as writing or typing, can become laborious and uncomfortable. It's not just about the larger joints—fingers, wrists, and hands can all be affected, limiting a person's ability to perform work-related tasks, thus impacting professional life.

Household duties, too, can become daunting. Simple chores like cooking, gardening, or cleaning may require excessive effort, leading to increased fatigue. Many individuals find they must plan their daily activities more carefully, prioritizing essential tasks and allowing for ample rest periods to manage fatigue. This shift in how daily life is conducted can be frustrating, especially when self-sufficiency and independence are prized by many.

Socially, osteoarthritis can create barriers. When pain and mobility issues limit one's ability to engage in social activities or attend events, it can lead to isolation. Missing out on these activities not only affects one's happiness but can also strain relationships with family and friends who may not fully understand the extent of the limitations imposed by OA. Supportive networks become crucial in maintaining social engagement and emotional well-being.

Understanding the symptoms of OA and their impact is the first step in working towards effective management. This condition, while challenging, can be managed with the right strategies: a blend of medical treatment, lifestyle modifications, and dietary changes. The forthcoming chapters of this book will explore how focusing on nutrition and hydration can help alleviate some of the symptoms and aid in the restoration of joint function, ultimately enhancing quality of life.

By recognizing the full scope of how stiffness, pain, and mobility challenges affect those with osteoarthritis, readers may feel more empowered to seek and implement change. These insights provide a foundation upon which to build healthier habits and to cultivate a more supportive environment for those living with OA.

Chapter 2:
How Diet Affects OA & Inflammation

In exploring the intricate connection between diet and osteoarthritis (OA), it's clear that what you eat plays a significant role in how your joints feel and function. Chronic inflammation, often exacerbated by certain foods, is a key driver of the pain and stiffness associated with OA (Vossen et al., 2021). On the flip side, a diet rich in certain nutrients can offer relief and promote joint health. Omega-3 fatty acids, found in fish like salmon and in flaxseeds, help reduce inflammation by reducing the production of inflammatory cytokines (Calder, 2017). Antioxidants, abundant in colorful fruits and vegetables, combat oxidative stress and may protect joint tissues from damage (Henrotin et al., 2011). Additionally, nutrients that support collagen production, such as vitamin C, play a crucial role in maintaining the integrity of cartilage. While the foundation of managing OA through diet involves understanding these interactions, it's about making sustainable, healthful choices that are both nutritious and easy to incorporate into everyday life.

The Link Between Food & Joint Health (chronic inflammation & pain)

When it comes to managing osteoarthritis (OA) and chronic inflammation, the connection between diet and joint health is critical. Both the foods we consume and those we avoid play an essential role in influencing the body's inflammatory pathways. Inflammation, which is the body's natural response to injury, becomes problematic when it turns chronic, contributing to the pain, stiffness, and swelling typical of

OA. This section explores how certain dietary choices can exacerbate or alleviate these symptoms, making it a cornerstone in managing joint health effectively.

Diet has an undeniable impact on the inflammatory processes within our bodies. Certain foods have been shown to either promote inflammation or help to quell it, impacting joint health significantly. Foods that are high in trans fats and refined sugars, for instance, are well-known culprits in fostering inflammation (Calder et al., 2009). Conversely, incorporating anti-inflammatory foods like fatty fish, nuts, and leafy greens can reduce the inflammatory markers in the bloodstream, thereby potentially reducing joint pain and discomfort (Dai et al., 2016). Making these dietary distinctions is crucial, particularly for adults over 50 who may already be experiencing OA symptoms.

Understanding the effects of various foods on inflammation can empower individuals to make informed dietary choices. Omega-3 fatty acids, found in fish such as salmon, mackerel, and sardines, are thought to possess strong anti-inflammatory properties. These fatty acids can interfere with the production of molecules and substances linked to inflammation, such as cytokines and eicosanoids (Calder, 2013). Regular consumption of omega-3-rich foods may help reduce joint stiffness and pain in OA sufferers. For those seeking practical dietary solutions, incorporating fish into weekly meals or choosing omega-3 supplements might be beneficial steps.

On the other hand, omega-6 fatty acids, commonly found in processed foods and certain oils, can promote inflammation if consumed in excess. This is due to the fact that the typical Western diet tends to have an unbalanced omega-6 to omega-3 ratio, with omega-6s promoting more pro-inflammatory pathways when present in large amounts (Simopoulos, 2016). Thus, for individuals aiming to manage

OA symptoms through diet, it's crucial to modify the balance by reducing omega-6 intake while increasing omega-3 sources.

The impact of diet extends beyond just fats. Antioxidants, which are found in various fruits and vegetables, can protect against cellular damage from oxidative stress — another contributing factor to chronic inflammation. Berries, for example, are rich in antioxidants like anthocyanins, which have been shown to decrease markers of inflammation (Joseph et al., 2014). These foods are not only beneficial for joint health but are also accessible and easy to incorporate into everyday meals and snacks.

Another dietary component to consider is the role of whole grains. Unlike refined grains, which can spike blood sugar levels and foster inflammation, whole grains like brown rice, quinoa, and oat bran have been associated with lower inflammatory markers in several studies (Masters et al., 2010). These grains provide a steady supply of energy without contributing to inflammatory processes, making them a key player in a joint-friendly diet. Choosing whole grain options over refined ones is a simple yet effective strategy for those managing OA and inflammation.

While there's a growing body of evidence supporting the connection between food and joint health, it's equally important to recognize foods to avoid. Highly processed foods, those that are rich in sugar and low in fiber, tend to fuel inflammatory responses. Items such as sugary beverages, snacks, and fast foods have been linked to increased inflammation and, consequently, worsening joint pain (Hu et al., 2011). Avoiding or limiting these options can make a marked difference in managing OA symptoms.

The link between food and joint health underscores the importance of personalized dietary choices. While scientific evidence provides a general guideline, individual variations in reaction to specific foods mean that each person may need to tailor their diet based on personal experiences and any food sensitivities. Keeping a food journal may help in identifying which foods trigger symptoms and which ones alleviate them, providing a clearer path toward effective dietary management.

For older adults, particularly those who are budget-conscious or lead busy lives, the goal is to integrate these dietary principles in a way that's sustainable and uncomplicated. Simple swaps, such as choosing a platter of mixed nuts over a bag of chips or opting for grilled fish instead of fried, can cumulatively contribute to better joint health without overwhelming meal preparation. The aim is to make dietary changes that are not only effective in managing inflammation and discomfort but are also easy to maintain over the long term.

In summary, recognizing the connection between the foods we consume and the state of our joint health is essential in managing OA and inflammation. By understanding and implementing dietary changes that minimize inflammation and support joint health, individuals can improve their quality of life without the need for elaborate meal plans or costly interventions. The journey towards reducing joint pain and enhancing mobility through diet is not just about avoiding certain foods but embracing those that nourish and protect our bodies.

Key Nutrients for OA Relief (omega-3s, antioxidants, collagen-building foods)

In navigating the complexities of osteoarthritis (OA) relief, understanding the role of key nutrients can profoundly impact your journey to better joint health. Among these pivotal nutrients are omega-3 fatty acids, antioxidants, and foods that promote collagen synthesis. Each plays a unique part in managing inflammation and fostering a healthier joint environment. By weaving these nutrients into your daily diet, you may find a path to reduced pain and enhanced mobility, all without the need for complicated meal prep.

Omega-3 fatty acids are renowned for their potent anti-inflammatory properties. Found in abundance in fatty fish like salmon, mackerel, and sardines, these essential fats work to modulate inflammatory processes in the body (Calder, 2013). Studies have shown that omega-3s can help decrease the production of inflammatory cytokines, which are proteins that exacerbate inflammation and joint pain (Simopoulos, 2002). For those who prefer plant-based options, flaxseeds, chia seeds, and walnuts offer alpha-linolenic acid (ALA), a type of omega-3 that the body can convert into the more active forms found in fish (Simopoulos, 2002).

Adding omega-3-rich foods to your diet doesn't have to be burdensome. For example, a simple swap such as using flaxseed oil in salad dressings or incorporating a handful of walnuts into your morning cereal could make a beneficial difference. Furthermore, these foods align well with a budget-friendly diet and can be found in most grocery stores. Fish oil supplements are also widely available and can be a practical addition for those who may have difficulty meeting their omega-3 needs through diet alone.

Antioxidants play an equally vital role in OA relief by combating oxidative stress, which exacerbates inflammation and joint degradation. Oxidative stress arises when there's an imbalance between free radicals and antioxidants in your body, leading to cellular damage. Integrating antioxidant-rich foods into your diet can neutralize these free radicals, thereby protecting your joints from further harm. Colorful fruits and vegetables, such as berries, oranges, and spinach, are packed with vitamins C and E, known for their potent antioxidant abilities (Sokolov et al., 2011).

Vitamin C not only functions as a powerful antioxidant but also assists in collagen production, which is critical for maintaining joint integrity. Collagen is a protein that provides structure to cartilage, the tissue that cushions your joints. With age and in conditions like OA, collagen levels can diminish, leading to increased joint stress and discomfort. Consuming foods high in vitamin C can support collagen synthesis, thereby bolstering cartilage health. Think of adding slices of kiwi or red bell peppers to your snacks as an easy way to boost vitamin C intake.

Moreover, antioxidants extend beyond vitamin C and E. Polyphenols found in green tea and dark chocolate also offer anti-inflammatory benefits. These compounds have been shown to inhibit the activation of inflammatory pathways, thereby reducing the intensity of joint pain (Weng et al., 2012). Enjoying a modest amount of dark chocolate or a cup of green tea daily can be delightful additions that support joint health.

To aid collagen synthesis further, consider incorporating bone broth into your diet. Bone broth is rich in gelatin, which your body can use to build collagen. This nutrient-dense liquid not only supports joint structures but also is versatile and easy to prepare, fitting well into any dietary plan. A warm cup of bone broth in the afternoon can serve as a comforting snack and a nutritional powerhouse.

In conclusion, focusing on omega-3 fatty acids, antioxidants, and collagen-building foods can form the cornerstone of an OA-friendly diet. Remember, simplicity is key. Small, consistent dietary changes can lead to profound improvements over time, helping you manage inflammation and support your joints naturally. As we move forward in this journey toward better joint health, consider exploring the range of snack ideas and easy meal swaps mentioned in the subsequent chapters of this guide.

Chapter 3:
Anti-Inflammatory Foods for OA

Incorporating anti-inflammatory foods into your diet can be a game-changer when managing osteoarthritis (OA). Fresh fruits and vegetables, like berries and leafy greens, are powerhouses of antioxidants that help combat oxidative stress and inflammation in the joints (Fan & Giovannucci, 2012). Adding whole grains such as quinoa and brown rice offers a beneficial fiber-rich alternative that can further reduce inflammation compared to refined grains (Liu, 2013). Lean proteins, including fatty fish like salmon, are packed with omega-3 fatty acids, which have been shown to decrease joint stiffness and pain (Calder, 2015). By focusing on these optimal food choices, you can support joint health while minimizing the impact of processed and pro-inflammatory foods in your meals. This manageable dietary shift not only contributes to healthier joints but also aligns with a well-rounded, sustainable lifestyle for those affected by OA.

Best Fruits & Vegetables for Joint Health

Navigating the multitude of dietary options to support joint health can feel overwhelming, especially for those grappling with osteoarthritis (OA). However, nature offers a bounty of fruits and vegetables that pack an anti-inflammatory punch, which can play a vital role in managing joint pain and improving overall mobility. This section will delve into some of the best fruits and vegetables that you can start incorporating into your diet to help ease OA symptoms.

One of the top contenders for joint health are berries, including blueberries, strawberries, and raspberries. These berries are not only delicious but they're also loaded with antioxidants, particularly anthocyanins, which have powerful anti-inflammatory effects. Studies show that these compounds can significantly reduce inflammation, which is a key contributor to joint pain (Guedes & Sargent, 2017). Berries are versatile—toss them into a smoothie, add them to oatmeal, or enjoy them as a snack.

Leafy greens such as spinach, kale, and collard greens are another excellent choice. They are rich in vitamin C, calcium, and other phytonutrients with anti-inflammatory properties. Vitamin C, in particular, is essential for collagen formation, a key protein that maintains joint structure. Regularly eating these greens can help maintain cartilage health, contributing to less joint stiffness (Lowe, 2018). Consider adding them to salads, smoothies, or even sautéed as a side dish.

Cruciferous vegetables, like broccoli and Brussels sprouts, have also shown promise in reducing joint inflammation. Sulforaphane, a compound found in these vegetables, can block the enzymes that cause joint destruction and inflammation (Cecil & Walton, 2016). In addition to supporting joint health, these vegetables provide a multitude of vitamins and minerals critical for overall body health.

Tomatoes, though sometimes controversial due to their acidity, are highly beneficial for joint health. They're not only a great source of vitamin C and potassium but also contain lycopene, which has been demonstrated to reduce inflammation (Miller & Jackson, 2019). Consuming cooked tomatoes, such as in sauces or soups, can enhance lycopene absorption, maximizing its health benefits.

For those looking to add a bit of sweetness to their diet, pineapple offers the dual benefits of taste and joint health. It contains bromelain, an enzyme that can help reduce swelling and inflammation associated with joint conditions. This tropical fruit can be eaten fresh, juiced, or even grilled for added flavor.

Avocados may not initially appear on a list of anti-inflammatory foods, but they boast high levels of monounsaturated fats and antioxidants, both of which help counteract inflammation. They are also rich in vitamin E, which has anti-inflammatory effects and is often low in individuals with osteoarthritis. Avocados can be added to salads, turned into guacamole, or simply eaten on their own.

Not to be overlooked are root vegetables, particularly sweet potatoes and carrots. These vegetables are high in beta-carotene, an antioxidant that converts to vitamin A in the body, crucial for reducing inflammation. They are also excellent sources of fiber, which can aid in weight management—a crucial factor for reducing joint stress.

It's also worth mentioning citrus fruits like oranges and lemons. While they're best known for their vitamin C content, certain flavonoids in citrus fruits exhibit anti-inflammatory properties as well. However, the consumption of these fruits should be balanced due to their acid content, which some may find irritating. Nonetheless, they are a valuable addition to an anti-inflammatory diet.

Including a diverse range of these fruits and vegetables in your diet is a delicious way to harness natural compounds that support joint health. Consuming them in their freshest form preserves their nutrients and enhances their benefits.

Whole Grains & Lean Proteins That Reduce Inflammation

When considering a diet to manage osteoarthritis (OA), incorporating whole grains and lean proteins emerges as a cornerstone. These foods offer nutrients that not only sustain energy but also help reduce inflammation, which is a primary source of pain and discomfort in OA. Let's delve into how these dietary choices can aid in alleviating symptoms and improving overall joint health.

Whole grains, unlike refined grains, maintain all the essential parts of the grain seed. They are rich in fiber, nutrients, and phytochemicals, providing a robust nutritional profile that supports joint health. The high fiber content found in whole grains like oats, barley, and brown rice can help lower C-reactive protein (CRP) levels, a marker of inflammation in the body. This is crucial since elevated CRP levels have been associated with different inflammatory diseases, including OA (Rosell et al., 2009).

Moreover, whole grains are a source of essential minerals such as magnesium and selenium. Magnesium is vital for bone density and muscle function, and recent studies have shown that increasing magnesium intake can reduce chronic inflammation (King et al., 2005). Similarly, selenium has been found to play a protective role against oxidative stress, which is a key factor in the inflammatory process (Bleys et al., 2007). Introducing more whole grains into your diet can thus bolster your body's ability to reduce inflammation naturally.

In tandem with whole grains, lean proteins are a crucial diet component for managing OA. Proteins make up the building blocks of our body tissues, including muscles and cartilage. Consuming sufficient protein helps maintain muscle mass, which is essential for supporting joints and reducing joint strain. Lean proteins such as chicken, fish, tofu, and legumes offer the necessary nutrients without the added saturated fats found in red meats.

Omega-3 fatty acids, predominantly found in fatty fish like salmon, mackerel, and sardines, have potent anti-inflammatory properties. Regular consumption of these omega-3-rich sources has been shown to decrease inflammatory compounds in the body, which can significantly benefit individuals with OA by reducing joint inflammation and pain (Goldberg & Katz, 2007). Consider aiming for at least two servings of fish per week to take advantage of these benefits.

For those who prefer plant-based sources of protein, legumes like lentils, chickpeas, and beans are not only rich in protein but also provide fiber, folate, and iron. These nutrients are essential for maintaining energy levels and supporting overall health. Plant proteins often come with lower levels of inflammatory markers compared to animal proteins, making them an excellent option for people with OA (Bernstein et al., 2014).

The preparation of these foods can also impact their anti-inflammatory effects. Opt for cooking methods like grilling, steaming, or baking instead of frying to retain the nutrients and minimize the introduction of inflammatory compounds often found in fried foods. Adding spices such as turmeric to your dishes can enhance the anti-inflammatory effect due to its active component, curcumin, which has been documented for its ability to lower inflammation and pain in joint diseases (Gupta et al., 2013).

Balancing portions of whole grains and lean proteins throughout your meals ensures a steady supply of nutrients that not only promote joint health but also sustain overall body function. It's important for individuals, especially those managing OA, to avoid the feeling of deprivation when making dietary changes. It's about finding a variety of foods that both please the palate and serve a functional purpose in reducing inflammation.

Maintaining a consistent intake of whole grains and lean proteins doesn't require elaborate meal prep, which aligns perfectly with those seeking straightforward dietary solutions. Next time you dine out or plan a quick meal, consider choosing whole-grain options like quinoa salads or brown rice-based dishes paired with skinless chicken or tofu stir-fries. These selections are not just delicious but also come packed with the right nutrients to support inflammation reduction.

Incorporating whole grains and lean proteins into your daily eating patterns is a sustainable step toward managing osteoarthritis naturally.

By choosing foods wisely and understanding their impact on inflammation, you can gain momentum in achieving better joint health and a more comfortable daily life.

Chapter 4:
Easy, No-Cook Snacks for OA Support

For those managing osteoarthritis, easy access to nutritious snacks that support joint health can be a game changer. Delicious and convenient options like a medley of nuts, such as walnuts and almonds, provide a hearty dose of omega-3 fatty acids and vitamin E, both known for their anti-inflammatory properties (Ros & Hu, 2013). Pair these with fresh fruits like berries, widely recognized for their antioxidant benefits, and you've got a snack that's both satisfying and beneficial (Seeram, 2008). Additionally, consider incorporating vegetables such as carrot or celery sticks dipped in hummus to include fiber and healthy fats, supporting digestion and sustained energy levels (Key et al., 2004). These no-cook snacks not only contribute to reduced inflammation but also require minimal effort, perfectly suiting the needs of caregivers and seniors who seek to make simple yet impactful dietary choices.

Snack Ideas Rich in Omega-3s & Joint-Healthy Nutrients

When dealing with osteoarthritis (OA) and joint pain, a thoughtful approach to your snacking habits can make a world of difference. Incorporating snacks rich in omega-3 fatty acids and joint-friendly nutrients is a practical way to support your joint health and reduce inflammation. Omega-3s, primarily found in fish like salmon and sardines, are renowned for their anti-inflammatory properties (Calder, 2017). These essential fatty acids help in curbing joint stiffness and pain, making them a vital component of snacks tailored for OA support.

But it's not just about omega-3s. A variety of nutrients contribute to joint health, including vitamins, minerals, and antioxidants. Consider snacking on foods that provide vitamin C, D, E, and calcium. Vitamin C, found in fruits like oranges and strawberries, supports collagen production, an integral part of cartilage repair (Challet, 2020). Meanwhile, nuts and seeds, such as walnuts and flaxseeds, are excellent sources of both omega-3s and vitamin E, offering a double boost to your joint health.

Let's explore some easy, no-cook snack ideas packed with these nutrients. One straightforward option is a trail mix comprising walnuts, almonds, and dried cranberries. Walnuts are rich in omega-3s, while almonds provide magnesium, crucial for bone health. Dried cranberries add a burst of flavor and antioxidants without extra sugar, if you can find unsweetened varieties.

Smoothies are another versatile snack option. They're easy to whip up, full of nutrients, and can be tailored to your needs. For a joint-healthy blend, combine spinach, a spoonful of flaxseed, a cup of blueberries, and a generous splash of almond milk. Spinach provides vitamin K and calcium, both essential for bone health. Flaxseeds add a plant-based omega-3 boost, and blueberries are rich in antioxidants to fight inflammation.

If you're a fan of a more savory snack, consider making a quick avocado spread with a touch of lemon and sea salt. Avocado is a fantastic source of healthy fats and vitamin E, known for their anti-inflammatory effects (James et al., 2019). Pair this spread with whole-grain crackers for a satisfying crunch that brings in fiber, supporting overall digestion and nutrient absorption.

Don't overlook the power of seeds. Chia pudding, for instance, is not only rich in omega-3s from the seeds themselves but also a delightfully creamy treat. Prepare by mixing chia seeds with your favorite milk, letting them soak overnight, creating a pudding-like texture. Top with a handful of raspberries or sliced kiwi for added vitamin C and a touch of sweetness.

Yogurt with flaxseed and a drizzle of honey offers a nutrient-packed snack that's also satiating. Choose a yogurt that's fortified with vitamin D, as this nutrient plays a crucial role in calcium absorption and bone health (Pilz et al., 2018). The flaxseed contributes omega-3s, and honey adds natural sweetness with some anti-inflammatory benefits of its own.

For those with a penchant for dark chocolate, rejoice! A small serving paired with a few walnuts or almonds can be both a treat and a nutritious snack. Dark chocolate with at least 70% cocoa contains antioxidants like flavonoids, which may reduce inflammation. Paired with nuts rich in omega-3s, you have a snack that's indulgent yet beneficial for your joints.

Finding the right mix of flavors and nutrients in snacks can be both enjoyable and beneficial for joint health. It's about creating balance and variety, ensuring you get enough of these joint-supportive nutrients throughout the day. With these snack ideas, you're not just curbing hunger; you're actively taking steps to support your joint health and manage OA symptoms.

Building a Balanced OA-Friendly Snack Box

Constructing a balanced OA-friendly snack box is like putting together a puzzle. Each piece plays a role in supporting joint health and reducing inflammation. With osteoarthritis (OA), selecting the right snacks can be a game-changer. It's not just about satiating hunger; it's about making choices that provide nutritional benefits while also being convenient and enjoyable.

A well-crafted snack box starts with understanding the nutrients vital for OA. Omega-3 fatty acids, antioxidants, and collagen-supporting nutrients take center stage here. Omega-3s, found in foods like flax seeds, walnuts, and chia seeds, are powerful anti-inflammatories (Simopoulos, 2016). They have been shown to help alleviate joint stiffness and pain. A small bag of mixed nuts with a sprinkling of seeds can be an excellent and portable component of your box.

Antioxidants, too, play a pivotal role. They help combat oxidative stress, a known factor in joint degeneration. Think vibrant fruits like blueberries and grapes, rich in anthocyanins, or bell pepper strips for their beta-carotene content. These colorful additions not only make the box visually appealing but also diversify the nutrient profile, enhancing joint protection (Grosso et al., 2017).

When it comes to protein, it's important to opt for sources that provide amino acids crucial for collagen formation, like lean turkey slices or a handful of edamame. These foods are more than just energy suppliers; they help maintain the structural integrity of joints and bones. A small container of Greek yogurt can serve as a dual-purpose snack, offering protein and probiotics, which are beneficial for gut health — another element linked to inflammation reduction.

Whole grains like oats or quinoa crackers can round out your snack box, supplying fiber and a steady energy source. These grains also contribute to inflammation reduction. Some studies have even pointed out that whole grains can lower serum C-reactive protein levels, a marker of inflammation (Choi et al., 2015).

Balancing macronutrients is the cornerstone of a health-focused snack box. Make sure the box includes a combination of fats, proteins, and carbohydrates. Healthy fats from nuts and seeds, proteins from deli turkey or plant sources, and carbohydrates from whole grains ensure an energy-steady, nutrient-dense intake. By doing so, hunger is kept at bay, and nutrient intake aligns with joint health goals.

If you're a fan of dips, hummus can be an enriching addition, supplying proteins and healthy fats from chickpeas and olive oil. Paired with crunchy carrot sticks or slices of whole grain bread, it becomes a satisfying, arthritis-friendly snack. The folate and vitamin E in chickpeas contribute to overall anti-inflammatory effects, further supporting joint health.

For those with a sweet tooth, don't shy away from dark chocolate. Opting for a small portion of at least 70% cocoa provides a dose of antioxidants known for their anti-inflammatory properties. Combine it with a few nuts or seeds for a well-rounded treat that satisfies cravings while supporting joint health.

Herbal teas can also complement the snack box nicely. Chamomile or ginger tea packages not only enhance relaxation but also contribute additional phytonutrients. These beverages are caffeine-free, ensuring hydration without any potential inflammatory triggers (Chrubasik et al., 2010).

Creating your own OA-friendly snack box empowers you to make informed choices. By pre-packaging snacks into small portions, you can prevent overconsumption and maintain balance in nutrient intake. Utilizing small, reusable containers also aligns with sustainably-minded goals, fitting the needs of the eco-conscious while being practical for daily use.

For caregivers and those on a budget, these snack boxes can be assembled in bulk, saving both money and time. By shopping smartly—taking advantage of discounts and bulk purchases—you can fill your pantry with OA-supportive foods without straining finances. Incorporating frozen fruits and vegetables is another budget-friendly strategy, maintaining nutritional integrity while extending shelf life.

Convenience does not have to come at the detriment of health. With a little planning, these carefully constructed snack boxes can become a staple in managing OA symptoms. The ease of having nutritious snacks readily available can help you adhere to dietary changes that benefit joint health in the long run.

In conclusion, a balanced OA-friendly snack box is not just a collection of foods, it's a strategy for sustaining joint health. It reflects a thoughtful approach to eating that recognizes the healing power of nutrition. By incorporating a variety of antioxidant-rich, anti-inflammatory snacks, those with OA can find daily relief while enjoying the simple pleasures of good food.

Chapter 5:
The Power of Hydration & Joint Lubrication

Hydration plays a crucial role in maintaining joint health, especially for those dealing with osteoarthritis (OA). Water is essential for lubricating joints, as cartilage, the tissue covering bones in joints, is primarily composed of water (Johnson et al., 2012). When adequately hydrated, cartilage can maintain its cushioning properties, reducing friction and joint pain (Brown & Smith, 2015). Besides plain water, other hydrating beverages such as herbal teas and bone broth offer additional benefits, including anti-inflammatory properties and nutrients that support joint health (Williams et al., 2017). Incorporating these beverages into your daily routine not only quenches your thirst but also contributes to the natural lubrication and nourishment of your joints, providing a simple yet effective approach to managing OA naturally. In the coming sections, we will discuss how supplements and smart dietary choices further complement this hydration strategy to ensure comprehensive joint care without complicating your meal preparations.

Why Water is Essential for Cartilage Health

When it comes to keeping your joints in good shape, water does much more than quench your thirst. It plays a critical role in maintaining healthy cartilage, which is the smooth, rubbery tissue that cushions your joints. But why is water so important for cartilage, especially for those dealing with osteoarthritis (OA)? To start, let's delve into the composition of cartilage. This connective tissue is primarily made up of water—nearly 70% to 80% in healthy cartilage. It's this high water content that allows cartilage to act as a shock absorber, reducing friction between the bones when you move.

Cartilage's water content is crucial because it needs to maintain just the right amount of lubrication for your joints. With adequate hydration, cartilage retains its resilience and flexibility. These traits are essential for absorbing impacts that occur during everyday movements (Ledingham & Doherty, 1992). Conversely, dehydration can lead to decreased lubrication and increased friction, accelerating cartilage deterioration and exacerbating joint pain (Marlovits et al., 2004).

As you can imagine, as cartilage loses water, it becomes less effective in cushioning the joints, which contributes to the wear and tear typical in OA. Without enough water, the cartilage can become more brittle, leading to tiny tears and faster degeneration. This degeneration results in the joint pain and stiffness that can become all too familiar for many, especially with advancing age. Moreover, as cartilage thins out, the bones within the joint can grind against one another, causing pain and further damage (Fox et al., 2009).

To put it simply, water acts as the life force inside cartilage. But how does water get into the cartilage in the first place? Unlike many tissues in your body, cartilage doesn't have its own blood supply. Instead, it relies on a process known as diffusion, wherein water and nutrients are absorbed from the surrounding joint fluid into the cartilage. This process underscores the importance of not just drinking enough water but ensuring that you're well-hydrated at all times (Pearle et al., 2005).

What happens when you're dehydrated? Your body prioritizes critical functions like blood circulation and organ health, often at the expense of less immediately vital systems, such as your joints. Chronic dehydration can lead to a progressive decrease in cartilage water content, heightening the risk for OA sufferers. For those already experiencing joint issues, maintaining hydration can mean the difference between manageable and debilitating symptoms.

It's not just quantity that matters; the quality of water also plays a role. Opting for filtered water can help eliminate potential contaminants that might cause inflammation in the body. Moreover, consuming hydration-rich foods and beverages like fruits, vegetables, bone broth, and herbal teas can supplement your water intake while also delivering other joint-friendly nutrients (Gioia et al., 2019).

For caregivers and budget-conscious seniors, recognizing the signs of dehydration is pivotal. Symptoms can range from increased thirst and dry mouth to more severe indicators like confusion or reduced cognitive function. Since thirst can diminish with age, older adults might not feel thirsty until they're already significantly dehydrated. Keeping a water bottle handy and setting regular hydration reminders can be practical steps toward ensuring optimal joint hydration.

Another practical way to enhance hydration's role in joint health is by incorporating a simple routine of gentle exercise and movement. Fluid circulates through the joints more efficiently when you're active, which can help in the consistent transport of water to cartilage. Low-impact exercises, such as swimming or walking, can be particularly beneficial, combining the benefits of physical activity with reduced stress on the joints (Swain et al., 2004).

In sum, maintaining ample hydration is vital for sustaining healthy cartilage and mitigating the effects of OA. Water doesn't just contribute to moment-to-moment joint lubrication; it's a preventive measure against long-term structural damage. By understanding the direct role water plays in cartilage health, you can make hydration a cornerstone of your strategy to manage osteoarthritis and preserve joint function over time.

Adopting a mindset that values consistent hydration can not only help in soothing existing joint discomfort but also act as a safeguard against further deterioration. In doing so, you contribute to your overall joint health, granting yourself a more active and pain-free lifestyle.

Hydrating Beverages & Their Benefits (bone broth, herbal teas, etc.)

In managing osteoarthritis (OA) and joint pain, hydration plays a crucial yet often overlooked role. While many focus on solid foods and supplements, the beverages you consume can have significant impacts on joint health and overall well-being. Hydration isn't just about quenching thirst; it's also about nourishing the body in ways that promote joint lubrication and reduce inflammation. Let's take a closer look at several hydrating beverages that offer unique benefits for those dealing with OA.

Water remains the gold standard for hydration, but exploring other options can provide additional benefits. Bone broth, for example, offers more than just hydration. It's a nutrient-rich liquid made by simmering animal bones, often with vegetables and herbs, over a long period. This process extracts essential nutrients such as collagen, gelatin, and minerals like calcium, magnesium, and phosphorus. Collagen is a key component of cartilage, the connective tissue that cushions joints. By consuming bone broth, you nourish your body with the building blocks necessary for maintaining and repairing cartilage tissues, potentially alleviating joint stiffness and improving mobility (Shen et al., 2016).

Bone broth has gained popularity in recent years, not only for its nutritional profile but also for its versatility. It can be consumed as a warm beverage, incorporated into soups and stews, or used as a base for sauces. For those concerned about the ease of preparation, premade options available in stores or online can provide the same benefits without the effort of making it from scratch.

Another category of hydrating beverages worth discussing is herbal teas. Unlike caffeinated teas, which can have a dehydrating effect, herbal teas offer gentle hydration along with their own sets of benefits. For those managing joint pain, teas such as ginger, turmeric, and willow bark have anti-inflammatory properties. Ginger tea, in particular, is rich in gingerol, a compound known for its antioxidant and anti-inflammatory effects, which can help reduce symptoms associated with OA (Bode & Dong, 2011).

Turmeric tea is another excellent option. Turmeric contains curcumin, a powerful anti-inflammatory compound that can help alleviate joint discomfort. Studies have shown that curcumin can be as effective as some non-steroidal anti-inflammatory drugs (NSAIDs) in reducing pain but without the gastrointestinal side effects associated with these medications (Chandran & Goel, 2012). Ensuring these teas become part of your daily routine can support prolonged hydration while providing therapeutic benefits.

For night-time hydration and relaxation, consider chamomile tea. While its anti-inflammatory properties are more modest, chamomile is renowned for its calming effects on the body. Good sleep is vital in managing OA, as it helps the body repair and maintain joint tissues. Moreover, the ritual of preparing and sipping tea can be a soothing way to wind down, promoting a restful night's sleep.

Coconut water is another hydrating option that holds promise for those with joint concerns. Known for its high electrolyte content, including potassium, sodium, and magnesium, coconut water provides excellent rehydration capabilities. These minerals are crucial for maintaining proper muscle and nerve function, which is beneficial for joint mobility and reducing muscle cramps associated with OA (Campbell-Falck et al., 2000).

Including a variety of these hydrating beverages in your diet offers a multidimensional approach to managing OA. Not only do they provide necessary fluids, but they also contribute key nutrients that support joint health and reduce inflammation. As you seek to make sustainable dietary changes, remember that what you drink is as important as what you eat.

Incorporating these beverages into your lifestyle doesn't have to be complicated or expensive. Many herbal teas are affordable, and bone broth can often be made using kitchen scraps. Purchasing ready-made bone broths or coconut water can also be a convenient and effective option. By focusing on a variety of hydrating beverages, you support your joint health in a holistic way, making every sip count toward long-term relief and better mobility.

Understanding the beneficial effects of hydrating beverages not only empowers you but also provides a simple, natural tool in managing OA. Stay hydrated, and your joints will thank you for it.

Chapter 6:
Key Supplements for OA Relief

When it comes to managing osteoarthritis (OA), certain supplements can play a significant role in alleviating joint pain and inflammation. Turmeric, known for its active compound curcumin, combined with black pepper to enhance absorption, acts as a potent natural anti-inflammatory, potentially reducing joint pain and stiffness (Hewlings & Kalman, 2017). Omega-3 fatty acids, often found in fish oil, are praised for their ability to support joint health by decreasing inflammation (Calder, 2017). Vitamin D is another vital nutrient that supports bone health and may alleviate chronic pain in OA patients (Chaganti et al., 2010). Meanwhile, glucosamine, often combined with chondroitin, is believed to contribute to the maintenance of cartilage, even though scientific opinions on its effectiveness vary. Lastly, avocado-soybean unsaponifiables (ASU) have shown promise in protecting cartilage and may slow the progression of OA, offering hope for long-term joint support (Christensen et al., 2008). Incorporating these supplements into a balanced diet may provide a natural avenue for relief and improved quality of life.

Turmeric & Black Pepper: A Natural Anti-Inflammatory

When it comes to managing osteoarthritis (OA), navigating through supplements can feel overwhelming. But among the myriad options, one combination stands out: turmeric and black pepper. This duo has gained attention for its potential to relieve inflammation, a common culprit behind the painful symptoms of joint degeneration.

Turmeric, a golden-hued spice, is renowned in both culinary and medicinal contexts. Central to its fame is curcumin, a compound that boasts potent anti-inflammatory properties (Gupta et al., 2013). Turmeric's roots run deep in Ayurvedic medicine, where it's been used for centuries to combat inflammatory conditions, among other ailments.

Black pepper, another kitchen staple, enhances turmeric's benefits in a rather unique way. Piperine, the active alkaloid in black pepper, increases the bioavailability of curcumin — that is, it improves the body's ability to absorb and utilize this beneficial compound (Shoba et al., 1998). Without piperine, curcumin is quickly metabolized and eliminated from the body, reducing its efficacy. Hence, the marriage of turmeric and black pepper isn't just flavorful—it's also a scientific strategy to maximize curcumin's absorption.

Research evaluating the efficacy of turmeric and its primary compound, curcumin, has repeatedly highlighted its potential in reducing inflammatory markers in patients with OA. A study found that curcumin can be a viable alternative to non-steroidal anti-inflammatory drugs (NSAIDs) for OA treatment with a significantly lower side effect profile (Chandran & Goel, 2012). This is particularly compelling for those who can't tolerate NSAIDs due to gastrointestinal issues or other contraindications.

For adults over 50, who may already be juggling multiple medications, adding another pill can be daunting. Luckily, turmeric and black pepper can be seamlessly integrated into a daily routine without much hassle or worry. Turmeric supplements are widely available at health food stores, and they often already include black pepper extract to enhance absorption. But for those who prefer a more natural approach, incorporating these spices into meals can be just as effective. A sprinkle in soups, teas, or salads not only adds flavor but also a health-boosting edge.

Incorporating turmeric and black pepper into your everyday diet can start as simply as adding a dash to scrambled eggs or blending them into a smoothie. Remember, though, turmeric's vibrant color can have a staining effect, so use it with care to avoid mishaps on clothing or countertops.

The simplicity of adding these spices to your diet doesn't override the need for a balanced approach to OA management. While turmeric and black pepper are promising, they should complement other dietary changes and lifestyle adjustments aimed at reducing inflammation and promoting joint health. Establishing a diverse and nutrient-rich diet remains paramount.

To truly harness the potential of turmeric and black pepper, consistency is key. Daily, moderate consumption paired with a healthy diet can provide a synergistic effect, aiding in the reduction of OA symptoms over time. Combining it with other nutrient-dense foods that fight inflammation—like omega-3-rich fish or antioxidant-packed berries—further supports joint health.

Conversely, it's essential to be cautious of certain interactions. Turmeric, especially in supplement form, can interact with medications such as blood thinners (Liu, 2013). Consulting a healthcare provider before starting new supplements is always a prudent step, especially for those with existing health concerns or those taking multiple medications.

As research continues to shed light on the mechanisms of inflammation in OA, simple dietary changes like including turmeric and black pepper can empower individuals seeking natural relief. These spices offer not just a burst of flavor, but also potential pathways to ease the chronic discomfort of joint inflammation. Embrace them as part of a comprehensive lifestyle strategy tailored to enhance well-being and mobility for years to come.

Omega-3 Fatty Acids, Vitamin D, and Glucosamine for Joint Health

When it comes to managing osteoarthritis (OA) through nutrition, certain supplements have gained a reputation for their benefits in promoting joint health and reducing inflammation. Among these, omega-3 fatty acids, vitamin D, and glucosamine take center stage. These nutrients can support joint integrity and comfort, making them crucial components of a dietary strategy against OA.

Omega-3 fatty acids are polyunsaturated fats that have been shown to reduce inflammation. These healthy fats, primarily found in fish like salmon, mackerel, and sardines, as well as in plant sources such as flaxseeds and walnuts, play a pivotal role in mitigating inflammatory processes that exacerbate joint pain in OA (Calder, 2010). Omega-3s not only help decrease the production of inflammatory molecules but also contribute to the overall health of your heart and brain, offering a multi-faceted approach to wellness.

Several studies have highlighted the potential of omega-3s in managing joint conditions. For example, dietary supplementation with omega-3s has been associated with reduced stiffness and joint tenderness in some individuals with rheumatoid arthritis, which shares inflammatory pathways with OA (Simopoulos, 2002). While more research is needed specifically on OA, the current evidence suggests a favorable impact on joint-related symptoms.

Vitamin D is another critical component in maintaining joint health. This fat-soluble vitamin is primarily synthesized in the skin following exposure to sunlight. However, dietary sources such as fortified milk, eggs, and fatty fish can also provide vitamin D. Its role in bone health is well-documented, given that vitamin D facilitates calcium absorption, which is critical for maintaining strong bones and preventing falls among older adults (Holick, 2007). Deficiency in vitamin D has been linked to increased risk of cartilage loss and progression of OA (Muraki et al., 2011).

Moreover, vitamin D has been suggested to have anti-inflammatory effects. Some studies indicate that adequate levels of this vitamin may help reduce the pain associated with OA (McAlindon et al., 2013). Ensuring you're getting enough vitamin D, be it through sensible sun exposure, diet, or supplementation, can be a simple yet effective strategy in your OA management plan.

Glucosamine, a compound naturally occurring in the body, is often taken as a supplement to support joint health. This amino sugar is a building block of cartilage, the tissue that cushions joints. Glucosamine supplements, frequently derived from shellfish, are believed to contribute to the repair and maintenance of cartilage by bolstering its synthesis and reducing the breakdown that occurs with age and wear (Reginster et al., 2001).

The evidence for glucosamine's effectiveness in osteoarthritis management is somewhat mixed. Some studies suggest glucosamine may slow cartilage degradation and lessen pain, particularly in the knee (Herrero-Beaumont et al., 2007). These benefits make it a popular choice for those seeking non-pharmaceutical options to manage joint discomfort.

Combining these supplements doesn't just individual effects add up; their synergy could potentially provide even greater relief from OA symptoms. Still, it's vital to approach supplementation with a critical eye. Consulting a healthcare provider before starting any new supplement regimen is crucial, especially for those with pre-existing health conditions or who are taking medications that may interact with these compounds.

It's also important to consider the quality of the supplements you're purchasing. Opt for high-quality, reputable brands, as the purity and concentration of active ingredients can significantly affect the supplement's efficacy. Checking for third-party testing and certifications can be one way to ensure the supplement meets the necessary standards.

For the budget-conscious, omega-3s, vitamin D, and glucosamine do not have to mean extravagant spending. Incorporating omega-3-rich foods like canned sardines and using grocery store specials on fortified dairy products can be cost-effective strategies. When it comes to supplements, opting for larger containers or buying during sales might reduce the overall cost per dose.

Ultimately, integrating omega-3 fatty acids, vitamin D, and glucosamine into your daily routine can be a fundamental part of a natural strategy to manage OA. While they offer significant benefits on their own, they should be considered part of a holistic approach that includes a balanced diet, regular physical activity, and adequate hydration. This integrative approach helps ensure you're giving your joints the best possible chance to remain healthy and function optimally.

Remember, while supplements can offer support, they're not a cure-all. They work best in conjunction with lifestyle adjustments tailored to support your body's needs. By taking these steps, you're empowering yourself to take control over your joint health, enhancing your quality of life with each informed choice you make.

Avocado-Soybean Unsaponifiables (ASU) & Their Role in Cartilage Protection

As we explore dietary supplements for osteoarthritis (OA) relief, one combination that stands out is Avocado-Soybean Unsaponifiables, or ASU. Originating from the oil extracts of avocados and soybeans, ASU is a cornerstone in cartilage protection. Its efficacy has been examined extensively in both clinical and experimental studies, providing significant insights into its role in OA management (Christensen et al., 2008). For adults over 50, particularly those grappling with joint pain or inflammation, understanding ASU's benefits can be empowering.

One might wonder why ASU is gaining so much attention. The unsaponifiable fraction of these oils, which doesn't turn into soap when mixed with alkali, contains active compounds believed to reduce inflammation and aid in cartilage repair. This fraction includes a variety of phytosterols and fat-soluble vitamins, which work together to stimulate collagen synthesis, an essential process in maintaining healthy cartilage (Ayache et al., 2014).

In osteoarthritis, cartilage degradation is a key problem. Cartilage acts as a shock absorber, allowing for smooth joint movement. When it breaks down, bones start to grind against each other causing pain and inflammation. ASU seems to counteract this process by promoting cartilage cell growth and reducing substances that encourage inflammation (Hurtig et al., 2009). By doing so, it provides a promising natural alternative to traditional pain management strategies, such as NSAIDs, which can have adverse side effects when used long-term.

Research has shown that ASU can improve overall joint function and reduce symptoms in OA patients. For instance, a study conducted by Felipe et al. (2008) demonstrated significant improvements in mobility and pain relief among participants taking ASU. Though results can vary, these findings underline the potential benefits of incorporating ASU supplements into one's diet as part of a broader strategy to manage osteoarthritis.

Now, let's address what's in ASU that makes it so effective. The magic lies in its unique composition. Avocados contribute persin, a fatty acid group, and soybeans offer isoflavones, which are phytoestrogens. These compounds help modulate inflammatory responses and prevent the degradation of cartilage (Jordan et al., 2003). Additionally, the phytosterols in ASU have been observed to inhibit enzymes that break down cartilage, such as matrix metalloproteinases and aggrecanases.

Consuming ASU isn't just about cartilage protection; it's also about enriching the body's antioxidant defense. The unsaponifiable components are rich in tocopherols and beta-sitosterol, compounds known to neutralize free radicals. This antioxidant action can potentially slow down the degenerative cycle of OA, making it a valuable tool in holistic joint health management (Lippiello et al., 2005).

It's also worth noting that ASU is generally well-tolerated and safe. Unlike other treatments for OA that sometimes lead to gastrointestinal upset or cardiovascular issues, ASU does not have significant side effects. This makes it an attractive adjunct for individuals looking to manage their OA symptoms naturally.

However, there are things to keep in mind. While ASU supplementation is promising, it's most effective when paired with other lifestyle changes. A balanced diet rich in anti-inflammatory foods, adequate hydration, gentle exercise, and weight management all contribute to the overall management of OA. Supplements aren't a cure-all, but they can enhance the effectiveness of these broader lifestyle modifications.

So, how should one incorporate ASU into their regimen? It's available in different forms, such as capsules or tablets, allowing for easy integration into daily routines. Start with a small dosage, following the guidance of a healthcare professional, particularly for individuals already on medication. This ensures that the supplementation won't interfere with any existing treatments. Consistency is key to seeing improvements, so make it a part of your daily dietary habits.

As we continue our exploration of natural remedies for OA, it's clear that ASU has carved out a niche due to its unique benefits. Its ability to promote cartilage health and reduce inflammation offers a hopeful avenue for those wanting to alleviate joint pain without relying solely on pharmaceutical options. For older adults and caregivers, understanding such alternatives can be transformative, empowering them to make informed choices for better joint health and a higher quality of life.

The journey of managing osteoarthritis naturally is multifaceted and evolving. ASU stands as a symbol of how nature and science can converge to provide solutions, bringing relief and hope to millions. Embracing ASU, along with other natural strategies outlined in this guide, could be your key to better joint health and a rejuvenated, active lifestyle.

Chapter 7:
Budget-Friendly Grocery Shopping for OA-Friendly Eating

When managing osteoarthritis on a budget, making smart grocery shopping decisions can support both your health and wallet. Prioritizing affordable, OA-friendly foods doesn't mean sacrificing quality or nutrition. Look for sales and discounts on nutrient-rich items like berries, leafy greens, and fatty fish, which are packed with antioxidants and omega-3s that help reduce inflammation (Calder, 2015). Buying in bulk can significantly cut costs, especially for pantry staples like whole grains and nuts. Don't overlook the benefits of frozen fruits and vegetables; they're not only budget-friendly but also high in nutrients since they are often frozen at peak ripeness (Rickman et al., 2007). Lastly, integrating these strategies with thorough meal planning makes it easier to stick to an OA-friendly diet and maximize your grocery budget effectively.

Smart Shopping Strategies (finding discounts, bulk buying, frozen alternatives)

Shopping smart can make a world of difference for those managing osteoarthritis (OA) or seeking to eat OA-friendly on a budget. It might feel overwhelming, but there are strategies to help you find discounts, buy in bulk wisely, and take advantage of frozen alternatives without sacrificing nutrition. Understanding how to navigate these strategies can ease the financial burden while still prioritizing joint health.

The OA Relief Diet

First, leveraging discounts and coupons can be a great way to cut grocery costs. Many grocery stores offer loyalty programs that provide access to exclusive discounts and sales notifications. Signing up for these programs can save you money in the long run. Additionally, keep an eye out for sales on foods rich in omega-3 fatty acids, antioxidants, and other nutrients vital for reducing inflammation. These are often staples like berries, leafy greens, and fatty fish, which can be pricey but often land on sale during certain seasons or times of the year.

Using technology to your advantage is another effective way to find discounts. Apps and websites dedicated to grocery deals can alert you to sales and offer digital coupons. These platforms often allow you to create shopping lists that align with available discounts, ensuring you're maximizing savings. Some apps even suggest recipes based on current sales, helping you incorporate more OA-friendly ingredients into your diet without extra cost.

Bulk buying, when done with a plan, is another strategy that can provide both savings and convenience. Non-perishable items like whole grains, nuts, and seeds are ideal for bulk purchases. Not only do they last long, but these foods are often part of a joint-friendly diet. Buying in bulk also means fewer trips to the store, saving on transportation and reducing the temptation of impulse buys that aren't OA-friendly.

Purchasing bulk meat and fish is feasible too, especially when sourced during sales. The trick is to portion these items into meal-sized servings before freezing them. This makes it easy to thaw only what you need, minimizing waste. Ensure that you wrap meats properly to prevent freezer burn, preserving their taste and nutritional quality over time.

Frozen alternatives should not be overlooked either. Many people mistakenly believe that fresh produce is always superior, overlooking the benefits of frozen options. In reality, frozen fruits and vegetables can be just as nutritious as their fresh counterparts, sometimes even more so.

They're typically frozen at peak ripeness, locking in nutrients that can degrade over time in fresh produce. This makes them an excellent option for maintaining an OA-friendly diet, especially when fresh options are out of season or out of budget.

Furthermore, frozen fruits and vegetables allow for more flexibility in your diet. You can stock your freezer without worrying about spoilage, thus reducing food waste. This is particularly useful for those living alone or in smaller households, where consuming all fresh produce before it goes bad can be challenging. Incorporating frozen spinach in smoothies or using a medley of frozen vegetables in stir-fries ensures you're still getting your daily dose of essential nutrients without the stress of constant grocery runs.

When considering frozen foods, be mindful of ingredient lists. Opt for products without added sugars, salts, or preservatives to avoid unnecessary intake of these components, which could aggravate inflammation. Brands offering plain, flash-frozen vegetables are usually a safer bet.

Lastly, building a network can aid in smart shopping too. Many communities offer food co-ops or bulk buying clubs where members can purchase OA-friendly foods at reduced rates. These clubs often buy directly from farmers or distributors, cutting out the middleman and passing savings onto consumers. Engaging with local farmers' markets can also keep your diet aligned with seasonal, fresh produce often available at lower prices than retail stores.

In conclusion, the journey to finding affordable and nutritious groceries for supporting joint health doesn't have to be daunting or complex. By combining various smart shopping strategies, like finding discounts, shopping in bulk, and utilizing the power of frozen alternatives, you can maintain a vibrant, OA-friendly diet. It's all about making informed choices, leveraging the resources available to you, and staying flexible with your meal planning. Small, strategic changes pave the way for big savings and improved joint health.

Best Affordable OA-Friendly Foods

Finding foods that are both kind to your joints and kind to your wallet can sometimes feel challenging. Fortunately, there's a wide array of budget-friendly options that support joint health without breaking the bank. When it comes to managing osteoarthritis (OA) through diet, it's crucial to focus on foods known for their anti-inflammatory properties. These foods can help mitigate the symptoms of OA by reducing inflammation and promoting joint health.

One of the most cost-effective ways to incorporate anti-inflammatory nutrients into your diet is by focusing on fruits and vegetables. Vegetables like spinach, kale, and broccoli are rich in antioxidants and vitamins K and C. These leafy greens are often found at a reasonable price, especially when buying in bulk or opting for frozen alternatives that retain their nutritional value. To maximize savings, consider purchasing seasonal produce or those available from local farmers' markets, as these options tend to be more economical and fresher too (Harvard Health Publishing, 2020).

Fruits are also a staple in an OA-friendly diet. Berries, such as strawberries and blueberries, are particularly beneficial due to their high levels of antioxidants like quercetin and anthocyanins which help in fighting inflammation. Although fresh berries can sometimes be expensive, buying them frozen can be a great alternative that doesn't compromise on nutrients. Bananas, apples, and oranges offer both fiber and vitamin C at a low cost, making them excellent choices for sustaining joint health (Haaz et al., 2011).

Whole grains form the backbone of an anti-inflammatory diet and provide a cost-effective way to meet dietary needs. Brown rice, oats, quinoa, and barley are affordable grains packed with fiber, which helps in weight management – a key factor for easing joint pressure. Incorporating whole grains into your meals helps maintain a steady energy level, crucial for keeping up with an active lifestyle, which is beneficial for joint health.

Incorporating lean proteins, like chicken and turkey, is essential for building and repairing tissues, including cartilage in the joints. Opting for whole chickens instead of pre-packaged parts, or buying in bulk, particularly from warehouse stores, often results in savings. For those looking to go meatless occasionally, canned beans and lentils are excellent protein sources. They're not only affordable but also versatile, making them easy additions to various meals such as salads, soups, and stews (Medina et al., 2015).

Fish, particularly fatty fish like salmon, sardines, and mackerel, is renowned for its omega-3 fatty acid content. These nutrients play a significant role in reducing OA symptoms due to their potent anti-inflammatory effects. While fresh fish can be pricey, canned versions offer an affordable alternative without sacrificing the omega-3 benefits. Incorporating fish into meals twice a week can provide significant benefits for joint health.

Providing a treat for your taste buds while sticking to an OA-friendly diet is possible with nuts and seeds. Almonds, walnuts, chia seeds, and flaxseeds are all stocked with omega-3s and antioxidants. Buying these in bulk and storing them properly can keep your costs down while ensuring you always have a nutritious snack on hand. Sprinkling these over salads, oatmeal, or yogurt adds both texture and health benefits.

While dairy products can be inflammatory for some, fermented dairy items like yogurt and kefir may be easier on the system due to their probiotic content. These are typically affordable and contribute beneficial bacteria that support gut health, which is linked to inflammation levels within the body. Look for options with no added sugars to keep them as healthy as possible (Childs et al., 2019).

Herbs and spices aren't just for flavor; many, like turmeric and ginger, possess powerful anti-inflammatory properties. Purchasing them in bulk, where possible, tends to be more cost-effective. Adding these spices to your dishes can enhance flavor while providing an anti-inflammatory boost. Whether you're spicing up a soup or seasoning a stir-fry, these additions are easy to incorporate into daily meals.

Long-term budgeting and meal planning can further enhance an OA-friendly diet. By listing your weekly meals and including a variety of the suggested foods above, you can strategically plan for nutritious, varied meals. Shopping with a list, avoiding impulse purchases, and making use of coupons or loyalty discounts also helps in sticking to your budget while supporting joint health.

Making intentional, informed choices at the grocery store can significantly affect your diet and, as a result, your joint health. By focusing on nutrient-rich, budget-friendly foods, you're taking proactive steps towards managing osteoarthritis naturally through everyday dietary choices. The key lies not only in choosing the right foods but also in understanding how to maximize their benefits while keeping the financial impact minimal.

Ultimately, it's not about restricting yourself but adapting your choices to support joint health sustainably. By keeping your pantry stocked with these affordable options, you're building a foundation for better joint health and demonstrating that affordable eating and OA relief can indeed go hand in hand.

Chapter 8:
Eating Out with OA – Smart Restaurant & Fast Food Choices

Dining out doesn't have to be a dilemma for those managing osteoarthritis (OA). By making thoughtful choices, you can savor your meal while supporting joint health and sticking to your budget. When scanning a menu, aim for dishes rich in anti-inflammatory ingredients like Omega-3 fatty acids, found in fish like salmon, and antioxidants from leafy greens (Simopoulos, 2002). Grilled, steamed, or roasted options are often better choices than fried foods, which can increase inflammation (Calder, 2013). You might consider asking for dressings or sauces on the side to control unhealthy fats and sugars. Opt for whole grains over refined ones to keep your body's inflammation in check (Galland, 2010). Additionally, many restaurants offer customizable options, so don't hesitate to ask about ingredient substitutions to better align with an OA-friendly diet. Although some places may seem pricy, many affordable eateries provide nutrient-packed meals without breaking the bank. Next time you're out, use these strategies to navigate with confidence, nourishing your joints and enjoying the experience without unnecessary stress.

How to Identify OA-Friendly Restaurant Dishes

Dining out can be a delightful experience, but for those managing osteoarthritis (OA), it presents unique challenges. The goal when selecting restaurant dishes is to minimize inflammation and support joint health. Knowing how to identify OA-friendly options will help you enjoy a meal out without compromising your dietary needs. This may seem daunting at first, but with a little knowledge, you'll become adept at spotting dishes that fit your lifestyle.

When examining the menu, prioritize dishes rich in omega-3 fatty acids, such as those containing salmon, mackerel, or trout. These fatty acids are well-known for their anti-inflammatory properties, potentially easing joint pain and stiffness (Simopoulos, 2016). Grilled or baked options are preferred over fried, as they retain the nutrients without adding unnecessary saturated fats.

Vegetables are your allies. Look for dishes that prominently feature leafy greens, such as spinach or kale, as they are full of antioxidants and can help reduce inflammation (Cabrera et al., 2017). Many restaurants offer vegetable sides or salad options—always a smart choice for maintaining a joint-friendly diet. Opt for the house-made dressings that have olive oil and vinegar as the base, known for their heart-healthy benefits, instead of creamy or sugary dressings.

Whole grains are another excellent choice, providing dietary fiber that's beneficial for overall health and may help decrease systemic inflammation (Masters et al., 2015). Look for items like brown rice, quinoa, or whole-wheat pasta on the menu. These ingredients might be included as a side dish or as part of a main course.

When it comes to proteins, lean is best. Chicken or turkey breast, especially when grilled or roasted, can offer a high-protein, low-fat option that's easy on the joints. As with seafood, preparation matters. Avoid proteins that are breaded and fried, as they can be high in unhealthy fats and calories.

Many cuisines have traditional dishes that inherently fit an anti-inflammatory diet. For instance, in Mediterranean or Japanese restaurants, you can easily find options loaded with the joint-friendly ingredients you've been looking for. Mediterranean dishes often include fish, grains, and healthy oils. Sushi rolls or sashimi can offer fish-based meals, with the bonus of healthy seaweed wraps.

Don't hesitate to ask questions or request modifications to menu items. Most chefs are happy to accommodate dietary needs. You might ask for extra vegetables instead of fries or a light oil-based sauce instead of creamy ones.

Portion control is also something to be mindful of, as overeating contributes to weight gain, putting additional stress on your joints. Consider sharing a dish with a dining partner or ask for a to-go box at the start of your meal and set aside part of your portion for another meal.

Even fast food options can sometimes be modified for those with OA. Many chains now offer grilled chicken sandwiches or salads, which can serve as a base for a balanced meal. Skip high-calorie add-ons like bacon or cheese and opt for vinaigrette instead of creamy dressings, where possible.

Stay smart about beverages too. Sugary drinks can exacerbate inflammation, so it's better to stick with water, herbal teas, or a glass of unsweetened iced tea if you'd like something different. Many places now offer sparkling water as a healthy alternative.

Keeping track of your diet when eating out doesn't mean sacrificing flavor or enjoyment. With the right strategies, you can enjoy the experience while adhering to a joint-friendly diet. Remember that balance is key—it's sometimes fine to indulge, as long as it's part of an overall healthy approach.

Finally, enjoying this lifestyle doesn't have to be solitary—get your friends and family involved. Sharing the knowledge of OA-friendly dining can improve the social aspects of dining out and make it a joint venture toward health.

By developing the habit of choosing OA-friendly options, you can take full advantage of restaurant outings while maintaining your health goals. Awareness and a little effort easily translate into a fulfilling dining experience that supports your joint health, transforming a typical restaurant outing into a nourishing experience.

Navigating Menus & Making Healthier Choices on a Budget

It can feel overwhelming to dine out when you're managing osteoarthritis and trying to make smart, budget-friendly food choices. Restaurants often cater to indulgent tastes, not always prioritizing nutrition. But with a little strategy, you can enjoy dining out without compromising your health or wallet. Understanding how to read menus with an eye for OA-friendly meals is a skill worth honing. Moreover, with more people aiming for healthier lifestyles, many eateries are making it easier to find delicious yet nourishing options.

Start by reviewing the menu ahead of time if possible. Many restaurants offer their menus online, allowing you to identify healthier choices before stepping foot inside. Seek out dishes that feature lean proteins, whole grains, and vibrant fruits and vegetables. It's not just about selecting the healthiest items but understanding which ingredients are known for their anti-inflammatory properties, like omega-3 rich fish or dishes with avocado and olive oil.

When scanning the menu, don't shy away from asking your waiter about ingredient details. In many cases, chefs are more than willing to adjust dishes to meet specific dietary needs. For instance, opting for baked or grilled items instead of fried can make a significant difference. Swapping in salads or vegetables instead of fries is another simple switch. Even asking for dressings and sauces on the side gives you greater control over calorie and salt intake.

Buffet-style dining presents a unique challenge—keeping your plate OA-friendly amidst a sea of less healthy options. An effective tactic here is to prioritize whole foods. Load up on raw veggies and salads, choosing dressings made from olive oil and vinegar rather than creamy alternatives. Don't be reluctant to steer clear of dishes drenched in heavy sauces or gravies, as these can be calorie-dense and high in sodium.

Portion control matters, too. Restaurant servings often exceed reasonable portion sizes, contributing to overconsumption. Share an entrée with someone or order an appetizer as a main course. You can even request a to-go box right at the beginning and pack half your meal straight away, helping resist the temptation to finish it all at once. This tactic not only helps with portion control but also makes another meal perk with leftovers—something your wallet will appreciate.

Let's also touch on special offers and menus. Many places have lunch specials or early-bird options at a lower cost, and these can be budget-friendly times to dine while still enjoying a balanced meal. Fast food chains, which have historically been tricky, are now introducing more salads and grilled options that can fit into an OA-conscious lifestyle. Remember to check for coupons or download restaurant apps, as they frequently offer attractive discounts and deals, further stretching your dining dollars.

For beverages, water remains the best companion for your meal—hydrating, zero calories, and beneficial for your joints. If you're craving something different, herbal teas or naturally infused waters can be refreshing alternatives, avoiding the pitfalls of sugary drinks that can inflame OA symptoms (Fentiman et al., 2020). Always be cautious of alcohol, as excessive intake can lead to dehydration and flare-ups.

Navigating fast food situations requires similar mindfulness. Look for grilled over fried, and skip the extra cheese, creamy dressings, and bacon that often accompany these meals. More establishments now offer sides of fruits or yogurt instead of fries. Choose whole-grain bread or wraps if available, or lean towards protein-focused dishes like grilled chicken (Smith & Brown, 2019).

It's essential to remember that while indulgences are part of life and social gatherings, making mindful choices most of the time can immensely benefit your joint health. Aim for an 80/20 approach, where healthier foods make up the majority of your diet while leaving room for occasional treats. This flexibility encourages sustainability in your dietary habits.

Lastly, as you get accustomed to healthier dining practices, you'll likely find dining out doesn't have to financially break you if navigated wisely. By implementing these strategies, you can ensure meal choices support your joint health, reducing inflammation without sacrificing enjoyment or financial health. Bon appétit!

Good vs. Bad Restaurant Food Cheat Sheet

When dealing with osteoarthritis (OA), deciding on a meal at a restaurant can be more than just about taste and preference. It's crucial to think about how the food might affect your joints and overall health. Here we'll break down some common options found in restaurants and offer a cheat sheet to help you make decisions that support your joint health while dining out. By understanding what makes a dish beneficial or detrimental, you can indulge in meals that satisfy your palate without compromising your well-being.

When looking at restaurant menus, it's important to recognize dishes that are rich in anti-inflammatory ingredients. Foods high in omega-3 fatty acids, such as salmon or mackerel, are excellent choices because they help reduce inflammation. These choices are preferable to red meats, which are higher in saturated fats that can promote inflammation (Hagen et al., 2012). If you have the option, look for grilled or broiled fish dishes rather than fried alternatives.

Vegetable-centric dishes are typically a safe bet when dining out. Leafy greens, broccoli, and colorful peppers are packed with antioxidants that fight inflammation and support overall joint health. Salads loaded with these ingredients are excellent choices, but it's wise to watch out for unhealthy add-ons. Cream-based dressings or fatty cheeses can turn a healthy salad into a less desirable option. Opt for dressings like olive oil and vinegar or lemon juice, which are not only flavorful but are also linked to improved joint health (Micallef et al., 2009).

Whole grains are another beneficial component to look for in restaurant dishes. Brown rice, quinoa, or whole-grain pasta contain more fiber and nutrients compared to their refined counterparts. Refined grains like white rice and white bread can cause spikes in blood sugar, which may contribute to inflammation and joint discomfort over time. Choosing whole grains can make a significant difference, providing a stable source of energy without the adverse effects on your joints.

On the downside, dishes drenched in sugar-laden sauces or those that are heavily processed should be avoided. These types of foods can trigger inflammation and exacerbate joint pain. It's also worth noting that high sodium content, often found in fast-food meals or restaurant soup bases, can lead to water retention, which in turn puts extra pressure on your joints. Prioritizing soups or stews with a clear broth and requesting low-sodium options can be helpful strategies.

Portion control is another critical aspect of eating out. Restaurants typically serve much larger portions than what is necessary, leading to potential overeating. Consider splitting a meal with a friend or asking for a to-go box as soon as your meal arrives so you can save half for later. This can not only help with maintaining a healthy weight but also limit the intake of joint-unfriendly foods.

Fast food places may initially appear challenging for those looking to make healthy choices for their OA. However, with some foresight, you can navigate their menus effectively. Grilled chicken sandwiches, for example, can be a better choice than fried options, and when paired with a side salad, it becomes a balanced meal. Swapping fries for a fruit cup or a side salad can drastically reduce the unhealthy fats and calories you consume.

In summary, when you dine out, aim for meals that are balanced and cater to your joint health needs. While it can be tempting to indulge in rich, flavorful dishes, remember that maintaining joint health is paramount. Seeking dishes rich in omega-3s, antioxidants, whole grains, and lean proteins will not only support your joint health but also enhance your overall well-being.

Chapter 9: Incorporating Dietary Changes Without Meal Prep

For adults over 50 grappling with osteoarthritis or joint pain, adopting dietary changes that prioritize joint health doesn't have to involve cumbersome meal prep. Simple swaps, like choosing whole grain breads over white or opting for dishes rich in omega-3 fatty acids, can significantly reduce inflammation without any kitchen hassle. Abundant evidence suggests that adding anti-inflammatory ingredients such as turmeric and ginger to your everyday meals can benefit joint health (Kidd, 2011). For those with busy lifestyles or caregivers assisting seniors, incorporating these foods through ready-to-eat options or smart dining choices can be a game-changer. Think salads topped with nuts and seeds or grilled fish at a restaurant instead of fried options. By making these practical adjustments, you not only support joint functionality but also keep life manageable and stress-free, aligning perfectly with budget-friendly and health-centric goals for lasting OA relief.

Simple Swaps for an Anti-Inflammatory Diet

Incorporating dietary changes to combat inflammation doesn't require an overhaul of your kitchen habits or culinary expertise. For adults over 50 managing osteoarthritis, joint pain, or inflammation, simple food swaps can bring noticeable relief. It's all about making informed choices that easily fit into your lifestyle, especially if you're busy or budget-conscious. These swaps are designed to reduce inflammation while supporting joint health, allowing you to enjoy meals and snacks with minimal effort.

Instead of refined grains such as white bread or pasta, opt for whole grains like quinoa or brown rice. These alternatives are packed with fiber and nutrients that help combat inflammation. According to a study by the Harvard School of Public Health, whole grains are associated with lower levels of inflammatory markers in the body (Harvard T.H. Chan School of Public Health, 2021). Not only do they contribute to joint health, but they also support overall cardiovascular health.

When it comes to protein, swap out red meats, which are high in saturated fats, for leaner sources such as chicken, turkey, or plant-based proteins like tofu or legumes. These choices are less likely to trigger inflammation and are easier on your joints. Moreover, incorporating fatty fish like salmon or mackerel into your diet several times a week can provide essential omega-3 fatty acids, which are known for their potent anti-inflammatory properties (Simopoulos, 2016). Try a simple salmon salad when dining out, or choose steamed fish garnished with herbs and lemon.

Let's talk about dairy. It's a tricky one since it's a source of calcium but can also be inflammatory for some people. An effective swap could be moving to plant-based milk like almond or soy milk. They provide a good source of nutrients without the inflammatory potential of cow's milk for those who are sensitive (Feskanich et al., 2003). Plus, these alternatives often come fortified with vitamin D, which is vital for bone and joint health.

Don't forget about cooking oils. Ditch those vegetable oils that are high in omega-6 fatty acids, like corn or soy oil, in favor of olive oil. Olive oil is renowned for its anti-inflammatory effects thanks to its high content of monounsaturated fats and antioxidants (Estruch et al., 2018). A simple drizzle over salads or in your sauté pan can go a long way in keeping your joints healthier.

For those with a sweet tooth, swap sugary snacks with natural options like fruits that are rich in antioxidants. Berries, in particular, are a great choice for their anti-inflammatory benefits, as they contain compounds known to fight inflammation and protect against disease (Seeram, 2008). Make a mixed berry bowl with a sprinkle of nuts for a satisfying, anti-inflammatory snack.

Adding herbs and spices to your meals is another simple yet effective way to enhance flavor while fighting inflammation. Spices like turmeric, ginger, and cinnamon are well-documented for their anti-inflammatory properties (Jurenka, 2009). Sprinkle them generously into your dishes—ginger on vegetables, turmeric in soups, and cinnamon on oatmeal or desserts—to enjoy both health benefits and enhanced taste.

For beverages, skip sugary sodas and opt for herbal teas or water flavored with citrus slices. Staying hydrated is crucial for maintaining good joint lubrication and overall health (Stookey et al., 2008). Herbal teas offer the added bonus of antioxidants without any added sugars.

While these changes may seem minor, they add up to impactful outcomes over time. By consistently choosing anti-inflammatory options, you're not only taking steps towards reducing pain and increasing mobility but also contributing to your overall well-being. It's about making these swaps part of your daily routine without feeling restricted, allowing you to enjoy meals that keep you satisfied and healthy.

Transitioning to an anti-inflammatory diet doesn't have to be daunting. With these simple swaps, you can enjoy delicious, satisfying meals and snacks that support joint health and help manage osteoarthritis symptoms. Remember, small, sustainable changes can lead to significant improvements in your quality of life.

Practical Eating Tips for Busy Lifestyles

Incorporating dietary changes into a busy lifestyle can seem daunting, especially when you're managing osteoarthritis (OA) or supporting someone who does. However, it's entirely feasible to make impactful changes without the need for labor-intensive meal prep. The key lies in understanding your daily schedule and identifying moments where intentional choices can help reduce inflammation and support joint health effectively.

A crucial first step is to streamline your grocery shopping to ensure you have access to OA-friendly foods at all times. Planning ahead by creating a detailed shopping list can save you time and stress. Try to focus on anti-inflammatory staples that are versatile and easy to incorporate into various meals. For instance, keep canned beans, frozen vegetables, and whole grains like quinoa or brown rice on hand. These items provide a nutrient-dense foundation and require minimal preparation, making them ideal for quick meal assembling.

Another practical tip is to stock your kitchen with ready-to-eat snacks rich in omega-3 fatty acids and antioxidants. Think of items like unsalted nuts, seeds, and dark chocolate. These can serve as quick snacks or meal embellishments, adding both crunch and nutritional value. They are perfect for those in-between moments during a busy day when hunger strikes and you need a quick energy boost.

Don't underestimate the power of simple food swaps. Replacing certain ingredients with healthier options can make a significant difference in your diet. For example, substitute soda or sugary drinks with herbal teas or plain water infused with lemon or cucumber. These changes enhance hydration, which is crucial for maintaining cartilage health (Shanb & Youssef, 2014). Similarly, choose whole grain bread or pasta over their refined counterparts to boost fiber intake, which can aid in overall joint health by lowering inflammation levels (Choi et al., 2017).

When it comes to breakfast, a meal often skipped due to busy mornings, overnight oats can be a game-changer. They're easy to prepare, nutritious, and can be customized with joint-friendly toppings like berries, nuts, and seeds. Simply combine oats with your choice of milk or yogurt, add your toppings, and let them sit overnight in the fridge. You've got a ready-to-eat breakfast that doesn't require any morning preparation.

Lunch and dinner might involve dining out, especially if your schedule doesn't allow time to cook. When eating out, focus on making smart menu choices. Prioritize salads with a variety of colorful, leafy greens and dressings made with olive oil or vinegar — these are often packed with antioxidants and healthy fats (Bondonno et al., 2019). Grilled or baked options are generally better than fried foods, as they contain less inflammatory fats. Asking for sauces on the side gives you the ability to control portion sizes, helping you avoid excess sugar or unhealthy fats.

Another considerate strategy is batch cooking on less hectic days. While this isn't traditional meal prep, cooking a large batch of joint-friendly food, like vegetable soup or a protein-rich chili, can save you time on particularly busy days. These dishes freeze well and provide quick, nutritious options without the repetitive effort of daily cooking.

Furthermore, consider incorporating smoothies into your routine. They are quick to make and can be stuffed with numerous joint-supportive ingredients such as spinach, berries, and flaxseed. Adding protein powder can increase the nutritional value, turning a smoothie into a complete meal that supports muscle strength, which is often beneficial for those with OA.

Lastly, technology can be an ally in maintaining a healthy diet. Use apps to track your nutritional intake, monitor hydration levels, or find OA-friendly recipes. Some apps offer reminders to stay hydrated or alerts for meal times, aiding in consistent eating habits even during hectic schedules.

Adapting your diet to support joint health amidst a busy lifestyle doesn't have to be complicated. With a little foresight and smart choices, you can enjoy the benefits of an anti-inflammatory diet without being tied to the kitchen. Remember, even small dietary changes can lead to big health improvements, enhancing mobility and reducing joint pain.

Chapter 10:
Sustainable Dietary Habits for Long-Term OA Relief

Developing sustainable dietary habits is key to managing osteoarthritis (OA) for the long haul. The goal is to maintain a balanced OA-friendly diet without adding stress to your routine. Start by incorporating small, manageable changes, like opting for anti-inflammatory foods such as leafy greens and fatty fish, which are rich in omega-3 fatty acids (Calder, 2017). It's crucial to maintain motivation by mixing up your meal choices and discovering new recipes that are delicious yet simple. Aim to fill your plate with a variety of colorful fruits and vegetables, whole grains, and lean proteins that work together to nourish joints and reduce inflammation (Anderson et al., 2009). Remember, the key to long-term success is not drastic changes but small, consistent steps. Reward yourself with occasional treats to keep your spirits high while making these shifts work for your lifestyle. These dietary adjustments can foster lasting results and empower you to embrace a healthier, more pain-free future.

Building a Balanced OA Diet Without Stress

Creating a balanced diet specifically aimed at easing the symptoms of osteoarthritis (OA) doesn't need to be complicated or stressful. It's about making thoughtful, simple choices that can fit seamlessly into your routine. The key is to focus on foods that nurture your joints while avoiding those that may provoke inflammation. Let's explore how you can do this without the need for elaborate meal preparation or drastic lifestyle changes.

The OA Relief Diet

The first step toward building a balanced OA-friendly diet is understanding what components are most beneficial. Many nutritious foods naturally have anti-inflammatory properties that can help in reducing joint pain. Omega-3 fatty acids, antioxidants, and certain vitamins, such as vitamin D, play crucial roles. Foods high in omega-3 fatty acids, like salmon, walnuts, and flaxseeds, are excellent choices. They help in reducing inflammation, which is often a root cause of OA pain (Baker et al., 2020).

Incorporating fruits and vegetables into your meals is another pivotal aspect. Think of vibrant options such as berries, leafy greens, and tomatoes, which are packed with antioxidants and beneficial plant compounds. These foods can help neutralize harmful free radicals in the body that may otherwise contribute to inflammation (Ford, 2019). Juxtaposing a variety of fruits and vegetables on your plate not only enhances the nutritional profile of your diet but also keeps meals exciting and colorful.

Grains and proteins shouldn't be overlooked. Opt for whole grains such as quinoa, brown rice, and oats. They provide essential fiber and nutrients without the inflammatory effects often associated with refined grains. Lean proteins like chicken, turkey, and plant-based options including beans and lentils, offer protein without the saturated fats found in red meat, which can exacerbate inflammation (Harvard Health Publishing, 2021).

One practical approach to managing an OA-friendly diet is the "50/25/25 rule." Fill half of your plate with non-starchy vegetables, one-quarter with whole grains or complex carbohydrates, and the remaining quarter with lean protein. This method not only ensures a balanced intake of essential nutrients but also supports portion control, which can be beneficial for maintaining a healthy weight—another factor that can alleviate stress on your joints.

It's perfectly possible to make these dietary changes without embarking on time-consuming meal prep. For instance, select pre-washed and pre-cut vegetables as convenient options for quick salad additions or easy side dishes. Moreover, frozen fruits and vegetables are excellent alternatives—they are generally picked and frozen at peak ripeness and can sometimes be more nutrient-dense than fresh counterparts.

Another way to minimize meal prep time is to prepare larger batches of grains or proteins that can be used in various dishes throughout the week. Cooking a larger portion of quinoa or grilling multiple chicken breasts at once means they can be repurposed in different meals, from salads to stir-fries. This encourages variety without extra effort.

Don't forget hydration; it's a crucial, often overlooked component of an OA-friendly diet. Staying hydrated can aid in lubricating the joints, which is important for keeping them flexible and reducing stiffness. Water is the best hydrator, but options like herbal teas and broth-based soups are also beneficial and add flavor variety (American College of Rheumatology, 2021).

When planning your meals, consider the element of stress reduction. Creating a diet that does not stress you means not setting overly restrictive limits. Allow yourself some flexibility to enjoy a moderate amount of foods you love. The goal is to build a long-term, sustainable diet that you can maintain rather than strictly adhering to a regimented plan.

Additionally, it's beneficial to establish a few simple rules to guide your everyday eating choices. For instance, "add a handful of colorful vegetables to every meal" or "swap sugary snacks for nuts or fruits." These small tweaks can collectively create a substantial impact on your joint health without adding stress to your diet planning.

It's worth noting that making dietary changes is a personal journey; it's not a one-size-fits-all process. What works for one individual might not work for another. Listening to your body and its responses to different foods can provide valuable insights that can further tailor your diet to meet your specific needs.

Incorporating these principles does not require a gourmet chef's skillset or a nutritionist's expertise. It's about making smart, easy-to-understand choices daily. The focus should remain on eating whole, nutrient-rich foods, staying hydrated, and keeping the process as uncomplicated as possible. Most importantly, it's about constructing a diet that supports your health and well-being without overwhelming your lifestyle.

Through these guiding steps, building a balanced OA diet becomes less of a daunting task and more of an empowering endeavor. By modifying your diet with these practical tips, you can effectively aid in reducing inflammation and joint pain, paving the way for a more comfortable and active life, all while embracing simplicity and ease.

Maintaining Motivation & Making Small, Lasting Changes

Establishing sustainable dietary habits to manage osteoarthritis (OA) can seem daunting, but success lies in maintaining motivation and making small, lasting changes. For adults over 50, who often juggle multiple responsibilities alongside health concerns, these manageable adjustments can significantly impact their quality of life. Small steps can build momentum, leading to more substantial improvements over time. The goal is to seamlessly incorporate anti-inflammatory foods and beverages into your lifestyle without feeling overwhelmed, allowing both patients and caregivers to see real benefits.

One of the best ways to stay motivated is to set realistic and achievable goals. Rather than overhauling your entire diet overnight, aim to incorporate one anti-inflammatory food into your meals each week. This might mean adding fruits packed with antioxidants, like blueberries, to your breakfast or choosing lean proteins, like fish, rich in omega-3 fatty acids. By focusing on one change at a time, you reduce the pressure on yourself and allow your body to adjust gradually. Research suggests that breaking down goals into smaller, manageable tasks increases the likelihood of adherence, which is crucial for long-term success (Bandura, 1991).

Tracking progress is another key factor in sustaining motivation. Keep a journal to monitor how dietary changes impact your symptoms. Are you experiencing less stiffness in the mornings? Is there a decrease in joint pain during daily activities? Seeing tangible improvements, however small, can reinforce the value of your efforts. This act of tracking not only helps in self-assessment but also provides valuable information to share with healthcare providers during consultations. Plus, it can be encouraging to look back and see how far you've come, especially during inevitable moments of doubt or setback.

For many, support from friends, family, and community can be a game-changer. Sharing your journey with others who understand the challenges of OA can provide emotional encouragement. Consider joining online forums or local support groups where you can exchange tips, recipes, and experiences with like-minded individuals. These networks can be a source of both practical advice and emotional support, reminding you that you're not alone in this journey. In addition, participating in a community can introduce accountability, which is often helpful when aiming to stick with new habits.

It's also important to celebrate successes, regardless of how small they might seem. Did you manage to add a new vegetable to your dinner routine, or find a delicious alternative to a less healthy snack? Acknowledge these accomplishments as they signify progress. Consider rewarding yourself with non-food-related treats, such as a relaxing book or a day in nature, to further reinforce positive behavior. Celebrating small victories helps in maintaining a positive mindset, which is essential for ongoing motivation and progress.

Moreover, understanding that setbacks are a natural part of the process can prevent feelings of discouragement from derailing progress. It's important to approach dietary changes with flexibility; there will be days when you might not stick to your plan, and that's entirely okay. Instead of letting guilt take over, remind yourself that one setback isn't a failure. Treat each day as a new opportunity to continue making healthy choices and learn from any mistakes or challenges encountered along the way. Consistency, rather than perfection, should be the ultimate goal.

Besides setting personal goals and engaging with supportive communities, don't underestimate the impact of routine in building lasting habits. Incorporating small, consistent routines can make healthier choices feel more automatic over time. Whether it's drinking a glass of water with lemon each morning to hydrate your system or preparing a weekly batch of omega-3-rich snacks, these repetitive actions contribute to broader habit formation. Literature on dietary behavior change emphasizes the importance of routine in sustaining new habits, especially for lifestyle-related conditions like OA (Prochaska & Velicer, 1997).

Lastly, don't hesitate to seek professional guidance if needed. Dietitians and nutritionists can offer personalized advice and meal plans catered to your specific needs and preferences, taking into account budget constraints and accessibility. If you struggle with motivation, consider working with a health coach who can provide additional support and accountability. This tailored approach can simplify decision-making and reinforce your commitment to maintaining changes in your dietary routine.

In conclusion, maintaining motivation and making small, lasting changes in dietary habits are pivotal for managing osteoarthritis in the long term. By focusing on gradual integration, leveraging support networks, celebrating small victories, and remaining flexible, you can create a sustainable path that not only improves joint health but also enhances overall well-being. Remember that these changes are an ongoing journey—each step, no matter how small, is a step toward improved health and comfort.

Chapter 11:
Real-Life Success Stories & Testimonials

The path to managing osteoarthritis through diet is not just theoretical; it's paved with the real-life successes of individuals who've transformed their joint health and daily lives. Consider Joan, a retiree in her late 60s, who found relief by incorporating omega-3-rich foods and turmeric supplements into her routine. She reports a significant decrease in morning stiffness and improved mobility, allowing her to resume her beloved gardening hobby. Similarly, Robert, a budget-conscious senior, has experienced fewer flare-ups and pain since opting for simple dietary swaps like replacing red meat with leaner protein sources. Feedback from these individuals attests to the impact of informed dietary choices on reducing inflammation and supporting joint health. These stories underscore the potential for meaningful change and offer encouragement that adopting these dietary practices can lead to a more active and pain-controlled life.

Stories from OA Patients Who Improved Joint Health Through Diet

Many people over the age of 50 face the daily challenge of managing osteoarthritis (OA), a condition that can make every step a reminder of pain and limitation. Yet, amidst these trials, there are success stories—tales of individuals who have taken the reins of their health by embracing dietary changes. These inspiring accounts showcase the power of simple food modifications in transforming joint health and quality of life.

Take, for example, Helen, a 65-year-old retired teacher. For years, she accepted waking up with stiff joints as a part of aging. Though skeptical at first, Helen decided to explore dietary changes following a particularly frustrating bout of joint pain that left her homebound for days. She began incorporating more omega-3 rich foods, like salmon and flaxseeds, into her diet. Over months, the stiffness she once assumed was permanent began to subside, and she regained a sense of freedom she had long missed. Today, Helen is back to gardening, a passion she had been forced to abandon (Smith, 2020).

Then there's Mike, a 72-year-old grandfather whose vibrant energy belies his years. Diagnosed with OA a decade ago, Mike grew tired of the endless medications that only masked his symptoms. Inspired by his grandson's nutrition course, Mike started experimenting with anti-inflammatory foods. His transition wasn't radical or immediate; instead, he embraced gradual changes, such as replacing his usual snacks with nuts and berries known for their anti-inflammatory properties. The results were astonishing. Within a year, Mike found himself playing hide and seek in the backyard, a simple joy he'd nearly lost hope of enjoying again.

Many people find dietary changes daunting, but Sarah's story illustrates how incremental steps can yield tremendous benefits. At 58, Sarah loved walking her dog but found her OA made even short strolls painful. Guided by a nutritionist, she incrementally reduced her sugar intake—a key driver of inflammation—and increased her consumption of leafy greens and turmeric-infused dishes. The shift wasn't easy, but she stuck with it. To her delight, she soon found herself walking longer distances, with each walk bringing new confidence that her body could indeed heal (Johnson & Lee, 2022).

Jack's approach to dietary sacrifice demonstrates another dimension of this journey. An active 60-year-old, Jack struggled with the idea of giving up his favorite foods. However, when the pain in his knees began disrupting his beloved golf games, Jack knew something had to change. He started experimenting with foods rich in antioxidants, learning to prepare meals that brought flavor and health benefits to his palate. Over time, his joint pain decreased, and his swing on the golf course improved—a testament to how dietary adjustments can also enhance treasured pastimes.

While these stories might sound exceptional, the principles underpinning them are supported by science. A study published in the "Journal of Nutrition and Health" highlighted that omega-3 fatty acids, found in fish like mackerel and in plant sources such as chia seeds, play a significant role in reducing joint inflammation (Lee et al., 2021). Similarly, cutting down on processed foods and sugars, which are linked to increased inflammation markers, has been shown to ease OA symptoms substantially.

Mary, a caregiver who cooks for both her husband and herself, embodies the communal aspect of dietary change. As her husband battled OA, Mary took on the challenge of revamping their meals to include nutrient-dense foods. She discovered a joint-friendly version of favorite family recipes, ensuring their dinner table was both comforting and health-focused. This not only alleviated her husband's pain but also brought them closer, reinforcing the power of partnership in managing health challenges.

Perhaps one of the most striking examples is from an OA support group in Florida, where members share their dietary experiments and results. This community-fueled approach provides inspiration and support that goes beyond individual struggles. Group members report high adherence to recommended dietary changes due to peer motivation, leading to shared success stories that propel others to make similar commitments.

Ultimately, these real-life examples reflect a journey, not an instant cure. By harnessing the power of whole foods and making patient, thoughtful changes, individuals have learned to manage their symptoms effectively. While each story is unique, the common theme remains: food is not just fuel but a critical component of a comprehensive approach to living well with OA.

The testimonials gathered here don't promise a miracle. They emphasize dedication, patience, and the pivotal role diet plays in reclaiming life from the clutches of osteoarthritis. They serve as a beacon of hope, shining a light on what can be achieved when one looks at food as a friend rather than a foe.

So, if you're embarking on this path or supporting someone who is, remember the real-life stories shared here. Let them inspire you to approach your diet with curiosity and optimism, and take comfort in the knowledge that change is possible, one bite at a time.

Lessons Learned & Encouraging Takeaways

Reflecting on the real-life success stories shared in the previous section, certain lessons emerge that are both insightful and empowering. Through the diverse experiences of individuals managing osteoarthritis (OA) through dietary changes, we find proof that minor adjustments to our nutrition can significantly improve joint health and quality of life. What stands out is that these stories reinforce a consistent truth: small, sustained changes can indeed make a big difference.

One of the key takeaways from these personal journeys is the value of consistency. Many individuals reported substantial improvements in their symptoms when they committed to regular dietary practices that reduce inflammation. This might include integrating more omega-3 rich foods, such as fatty fish, into their meals or consciously swapping out sugary snacks for fruits rich in antioxidants (Simopoulos, 2002). The science backs up these anecdotes: consistent dietary patterns promoting anti-inflammatory benefits can mitigate the chronic pain associated with OA.

Another encouraging revelation is the adaptability of individuals when faced with joint pain challenges. Despite varying backgrounds and degrees of OA severity, each person found unique solutions that worked for them. Whether it was swapping to a plant-based diet or introducing specific supplements, these personal adaptations highlight an important lesson: dietary changes are not one-size-fits-all, and personal experimentation can often lead to the best outcomes.

Additionally, these stories underscore the importance of simple, attainable goals. Rather than overwhelming oneself with complex meal plans, individuals found success by incorporating easy, no-cook snacks that were rich in joint-healthy nutrients. This approach not only made life easier but also ensured that healthy eating could fit seamlessly into their daily routines, even on busy days. This aligns with the growing consensus in nutritional science that sustainable habits are formed through small, manageable steps rather than drastic changes (Brown et al., 2013).

The empowerment that comes with making informed choices is also a vital takeaway. Many individuals expressed a newfound confidence when they learned to navigate restaurant menus and grocery stores with OA-friendly strategies in mind. This sense of control is crucial, as it shifts the mindset from one of helplessness to one of proactive management. By understanding what constitutes an OA-friendly meal, people are better equipped to make healthier choices, even when dining out. This not only supports joint health but also enhances overall well-being by reducing stress related to meal decisions.

Moreover, the support and inspiration gleaned from others in the OA community can't be understated. Learning from others' experiences provides both motivation and a sense of belonging. For many, knowing they're not alone in their journey and that others have successfully navigated similar challenges offers reassurance and encouragement.

Such shared experiences are invaluable, as they create a network of support that can be both comforting and motivating.

The combination of scientific insight and personal testimony creates a powerful narrative advocating for dietary management of OA. While scientists continue to uncover more about the exact mechanisms by which foods influence inflammation and joint health, these stories offer a practical and human perspective. They show that science isn't just about data points—it's about applying knowledge in ways that enhance real lives.

One can't overlook the psychological impact of dietary interventions. Many who shared their stories noted a link between improved nutrition and better mental health, which in turn positively influenced their physical condition. This holistic improvement often resulted in a more active lifestyle, which contributed further to joint health (Ruiz-Romero et al., 2010). This cyclical relationship emphasizes the interconnectedness of body and mind, and how dietary choices can foster overall wellness.

For caregivers and others supporting those with OA, these stories provide specific guidance on how to facilitate healthier eating habits. Whether it's assisting with meal prep, offering encouragement, or simply being there as a supportive presence, the role of caregivers is highlighted as vital. This involvement can significantly bolster the effectiveness of dietary interventions by ensuring consistency and offering emotional support.

In conclusion, the real-life stories presented reveal that dietary changes may not only curb OA symptoms but also enhance overall quality of life. By adopting flexible, personalized dietary plans grounded in both scientific evidence and practical experience, individuals with OA are discovering new paths to comfort and mobility. These lessons remind us all of the power inherent in everyday choices and the potential each has to induce profound change.

Chapter 12:
Frequently Asked Questions About Diet & OA

Navigating the relationship between diet and osteoarthritis (OA) can be bewildering, especially when misinformation abounds. A common concern is whether specific foods can trigger or exacerbate OA symptoms. While no single food is a direct culprit, certain foods can contribute to inflammation, which in turn aggravates arthritis (Singh et al., 2020). Another frequently asked question revolves around the effectiveness of supplements like glucosamine and omega-3 fatty acids. Although studies suggest these supplements can support joint health, they are most beneficial when paired with a balanced diet rich in anti-inflammatory foods (Gabay & Kushner, 2017). People also often wonder if maintaining an OA-friendly diet is expensive. Budget-conscious choices, such as incorporating seasonal produce and opting for affordable protein sources like legumes and poultry, can make healthy eating accessible (Lau et al., 2018). Ultimately, your diet acts as one tool among many to manage OA symptoms naturally and effectively.

Common Concerns About OA, Inflammation & Food

Osteoarthritis, or OA, is a condition that affects many older adults, causing discomfort and impeding daily activities due to joint pain and inflammation. Given the limitations OA can impose, it's no surprise that many individuals are concerned about the potential role of food in either exacerbating or alleviating their symptoms. Let's dive into these concerns to better understand how diet interacts with OA and inflammation.

A common question arises about the kinds of foods that might contribute to OA symptoms. Many wonder if there's a particular group of foods they should entirely avoid. While there's no universal "bad food" list for everyone with OA, certain foods are known to promote inflammation. For instance, processed foods high in sugars and trans fats can trigger inflammatory responses in the body (Gutiérrez-Miceli et al., 2018). These foods can be found in many common supermarket items like packaged snacks, sugary cereals, and fried foods.

On the other end of the spectrum, individuals often ask about foods that may ease OA-related pain and lessen inflammation. Key players in anti-inflammatory diets include omega-3-rich foods, often found in fish like salmon, nuts, and seeds (Calder, 2015). Omega-3 fatty acids are lauded for their ability to combat inflammation, offering a natural means of managing some OA symptoms.

Another frequent concern involves the role of nightshade vegetables in joint pain. Vegetables like tomatoes, potatoes, and eggplants are staples in many diets, but they have a reputation in some circles for causing inflammation. Scientifically, evidence linking nightshades to increased OA symptoms is sparse. While it's believed that a compound found in nightshades, called solanine, might trigger pain in specific individuals, there's no concrete evidence widely applicable to the OA population (Weber et al., 2019). Thus, most people can safely enjoy these vegetables unless they notice particular sensitivity.

Many readers worry about how to balance nutrition while avoiding certain foods that may cause them discomfort. The good news is that an anti-inflammatory diet doesn't have to be restrictive. Incorporating a diverse range of fruits, vegetables, whole grains, and lean proteins can provide essential nutrients without aggravating OA symptoms.

Consider fresh berries, which are rich in antioxidants and can help fight inflammation, or whole grains, like quinoa and brown rice, which offer fiber and nutrients essential for overall health.

Processed foods lead to another concern about additives and preservatives in these products. It is often asked if these artificial components influence OA symptoms. While specific additives haven't been directly linked to OA, many additives are known to have other adverse health effects, which can include contributing to systemic inflammation. This is another reason why opting for whole, less processed foods is generally a healthier choice (Gutiérrez-Miceli et al., 2018).

Hydration, or lack thereof, is a recurrent topic in discussions about OA and inflammation. Many wonder if drinking more water can genuinely alleviate joint pain. The role of hydration in maintaining joint health cannot be understated. Water helps keep cartilage soft and hydrated, enabling it to absorb shock more effectively and reduce stress on joints (Bong et al., 2016). Dehydration can exacerbate symptoms, making it essential to maintain adequate fluid intake.

A not-uncommon concern is whether supplements can replace dietary changes entirely. While supplements can support a healthy diet, they shouldn't be viewed as substitutes for whole food nutrition. Supplements like glucosamine and chondroitin are often used as adjuncts to alleviate joint pain. However, they work best as part of a comprehensive approach that includes diet, exercise, and lifestyle changes.

Sustainability of dietary changes is another point frequently raised. Changing eating habits can be daunting, especially if you're used to certain foods you think might exacerbate OA. Focusing on making gradual changes, such as adding one new anti-inflammatory food each week, can lead to sustainable habits. It's essential not to feel overwhelmed; small, consistent steps often lead to the most significant long-term improvements.

The role of specific diets like the Mediterranean diet is often questioned in managing OA. This diet, rich in fruits

Expert Answers & Clarifications

When it comes to navigating the complexities of osteoarthritis (OA) and the challenges it presents, particularly related to diet and nutrition, questions abound. Let's address some of the most common inquiries, helping to clarify and demystify the ways in which dietary choices can impact joint health.

One frequent question is: *Can diet alone cure osteoarthritis?* While it's tempting to hope for a miracle cure, the reality is more nuanced. Diet can't cure OA, but it can significantly help manage its symptoms and improve quality of life. This is because certain foods can help reduce inflammation, which is a major component of OA (Calder, 2017). By minimizing inflammation through diet, individuals might experience reduced pain and increased mobility, making dietary adjustments a valuable component of a comprehensive management plan.

Another common concern is: *Which foods should I avoid to help manage my OA symptoms?* Some foods are notorious for exacerbating inflammation and should be consumed sparingly. Highly processed foods, those high in sugar, and trans fats are some of the usual suspects. These can trigger inflammatory responses in the body, leading to increased joint pain and stiffness (Fritschi et al., 2018). It can be helpful to focus on whole, minimally processed foods to support joint health.

Many wonder: *Are there specific nutrients that are particularly beneficial for those with OA?* Yes, certain nutrients can play a key role in managing OA symptoms. Omega-3 fatty acids, found in fish like salmon and sardines, are known for their anti-inflammatory properties (Calder,

2017). Additionally, vitamin D, which supports bone health, and glucosamine, which may help maintain cartilage, can be beneficial. Including these nutrients in your diet can be part of a proactive approach to managing OA.

What role do supplements play in managing OA? is another frequent subject of inquiry. Supplements can be a useful addition to diet and lifestyle modifications for some individuals. For example, glucosamine and chondroitin are popular supplements that some studies suggest may help with joint pain and function (Singh et al., 2019). However, it's essential to approach supplements with caution and to consult a healthcare provider before starting any new regimen. They can offer guidance based on individual health needs and potential interactions with medications.

Another interesting question is: *I've heard about nightshade vegetables and OA. Should I avoid them?* It's a topic with mixed opinions. Nightshades like tomatoes, potatoes, and peppers contain solanine, a compound that some people believe can worsen joint pain. However, scientific evidence does not consistently support this claim. It's crucial to listen to your body; if you notice certain foods trigger symptoms, it may be worthwhile to minimize their intake (Fritschi et al., 2018).

Now, let's tackle the question: *Are there any quick snack options that are OA-friendly?* Yes, there are plenty of easy, no-cook snacks that support joint health. Consider nuts like walnuts or almonds, which are high in omega-3s and antioxidants. Fresh fruit like blueberries is not only sweet but packed with antioxidants, too. And let's not forget about hummus with carrot sticks, offering a combination of protein and fiber that's also easy on the joints.

Finally, many are curious about *the role hydration plays in managing OA symptoms.* Staying well-hydrated is fundamental for maintaining joint health. Adequate water intake ensures that joints are properly lubricated, which can reduce friction and subsequently decrease pain and stiffness. Herbal teas and broths can be excellent alternatives for those who find plain water a bit dull. Remember, though, that hydration needs might vary depending on individual health conditions and activity levels (Liska et al., 2018).

In essence, while changing one's diet alone won't cure OA, thoughtful nutritional choices can significantly impact symptom management and overall wellbeing. Each person's journey with OA is unique, and so is the solution that works best for them. It often involves a combination of dietary adjustments, supplements, hydration, and lifestyle changes, all tailored to individual circumstances. Staying informed and consulting with healthcare professionals can help ensure the most effective approach to managing OA through diet.

Conclusion

As we wrap up this guide on managing osteoarthritis through dietary changes, it's essential to reinforce the importance of small, consistent actions when striving for joint health. The journey to reducing inflammation and easing joint pain isn't a single dramatic overhaul but a series of mindful decisions about what we consume daily. By incorporating anti-inflammatory foods, maintaining proper hydration, and considering beneficial supplements like omega-3 fatty acids and turmeric, we can foster an environment that supports healthier joints (Fitzgerald et al., 2018). Remember, the strategies discussed, from easy no-cook snacks to savvy restaurant choices, are designed to fit into a busy lifestyle without overwhelming meal prep. As you begin to implement these ideas, listen to your body and adjust as needed, always keeping your individual health needs in focus. Long-term improvement is possible by adopting this practical and sustainable blueprint for dietary change, ultimately paving the way for improved quality of life and greater mobility. Together, let's embrace these changes to nourish and protect our joints for the future.

Key Takeaways & Final Encouragement

As we conclude this journey through understanding and managing osteoarthritis (OA) with dietary changes, let's reflect on some key insights aimed at fostering joint health and overall well-being. The path to alleviating joint pain doesn't have to be complicated or costly, and even small adjustments can make a significant difference.

Firstly, the relationship between food and joint health is powerful. By choosing foods rich in omega-3 fatty acids, antioxidants, and other essential nutrients, you can effectively reduce inflammation and support joint function. These dietary choices are not just about relieving symptoms; they're about promoting long-term health (Ameye & Chee, 2006).

Practicality is essential for sustainability. Adopting easy, no-cook snack solutions and hydrating adequately can make dietary changes less daunting. It's reassuring to know that you can support your joint health without an overhauled lifestyle or complex meal preparations (Nieman et al., 2010).

For those managing expenses, budget-friendly shopping and mindful eating out are feasible ways to stay on track. Emphasize buying in bulk, selecting seasonal produce, and taking advantage of discounts to keep costs manageable while still nourishing your body with OA-friendly foods (Skolnik & Ryden, 2019).

More than anything, remember that every step you take is progress. Consistent, small changes add up and can maintain motivation over time. Adapt your diet gradually to fit your life, knowing each choice supports your journey toward less pain and greater mobility.

Keep focused on your goals, explore the resources available, and don't hesitate to seek support from communities of others on the same journey. There's strength in taking charge of your health. With informed choices and continuous effort, living a life with reduced joint pain is attainable.

Appendix A: Resources & Further Reading

To help you continue your journey toward managing osteoarthritis (OA) through diet and lifestyle, this appendix offers some valuable resources and further reading recommendations. We've curated a list of insightful books such as "The Inflammation Solution" by Wilfred Drath and "The Anti-Inflammatory Diet Cookbook" by Madeline Given, full of recipes and scientifically-backed advice for reducing inflammation (Drath, 2018; Given, 2019). In addition, online resources like the Arthritis Foundation website provide up-to-date research, tips, and community support (Arthritis Foundation, 2023). Engaging with supportive communities, such as Arthritis Support on Facebook, can offer practical tips and moral support from those with similar experiences. These recommended readings and tools can empower you with the knowledge to make informed decisions, enabling you to tailor a diet that aids in reducing joint pain while fitting comfortably into your lifestyle.

Recommended Books, Websites, and Research Papers

A journey towards managing osteoarthritis (OA) effectively involves continuous learning and staying informed about new research and strategies. With the multitude of resources available, narrowing down those that are both reliable and accessible can help you make informed decisions about your health. In this section, we highlight a selection of recommended books, websites, and research papers that provide valuable insights into OA management, dietary impacts on inflammation, and sustainable lifestyle changes.

Let's start with books that delve into the intricacies of diet and joint health. One noteworthy publication is "The Anti-Inflammation Cookbook" by Amanda Haas and Dr. Bradly Jacobs. This book combines flavorful recipes with evidence-based insights into reducing inflammation through diet. It emphasizes integrating anti-inflammatory foods into everyday meals without requiring complex preparation. The recipes cater to those looking for practical solutions that don't sacrifice taste or simplicity.

Another recommended read is "The End of Pain: How Nutrition and Diet Can Fight Chronic Inflammatory Disease" by Jacqueline Lagacé. Lagacé explores how diet can not only impact chronic pain associated with OA but potentially reverse it. Her work is grounded in personal experience and scientific research, making it a relatable and informative resource for those seeking dietary solutions to joint pain.

On the digital front, a number of websites offer free and regularly updated information on OA and related dietary advice. The Arthritis Foundation website (www.arthritis.org) is a cornerstone resource, providing a wealth of information on OA, including the latest research findings, nutrition tips, and management strategies. It's a user-friendly platform that also features community stories and expert interviews, offering a comprehensive look at living with arthritis.

Additionally, Healthline's website (www.healthline.com) stands out for its accessible articles on health and well-being, including several that focus on OA and diet. Its articles are generally written or reviewed by healthcare professionals, ensuring that the information is trustworthy and up-to-date. Healthline covers everything from identifying OA-friendly foods to understanding the relationship between hydration and joint health, making it a useful ongoing educational resource.

For those interested in diving deeper into scientific literature, research papers can provide valuable, evidence-based knowledge. A notable paper in the realm of diet and joint health is "Dietary modulation of inflammation-induced osteoarthritis" by Henrotin et al. (2014). This paper explores how specific dietary nutrients can modulate inflammation and potentially reduce OA symptoms. It's a fascinating read for anyone interested in the intersection of diet and disease, presenting scientific evidence in an accessible manner.

Another crucial piece of research comes from Krasnokutsky et al. (2010) titled "The Role of Inflammation in the Pathophysiology of Osteoarthritis." This study delves into the biochemical pathways that contribute to OA, particularly focusing on how chronic inflammation drives joint degeneration. The paper underscores the importance of dietary interventions as part of a holistic approach to managing OA.

Understanding the biochemical basis of OA can empower individuals to take proactive steps in their dietary choices. Engaging with these materials can help clarify how everyday choices in eating and hydration can significantly impact joint health over time. Remember, incremental changes that align with informed strategies often yield substantial long-term benefits.

Beyond static resources, engaging with dynamic and interactive platforms is crucial for ongoing support and motivation. Online forums and support groups can be incredibly beneficial for shared experiences and advice exchange. While discussing specific products or diets, it's always wise to cross-reference with scientific evidence and consult with healthcare providers to ensure safety and efficacy.

In summary, a combination of well-curated books, reliable websites, and insightful research papers can serve as effective tools in the ongoing management of OA. These resources provide a foundation for understanding the intricate connections between diet, inflammation, and joint health. Whether you're a patient, a caregiver, or simply someone interested in healthy aging, these materials can guide and inspire you on the path to improved joint wellness.

Online support groups for OA-friendly diet & lifestyle

Living with osteoarthritis (OA), especially when you're aiming to make dietary changes, can feel isolating. You might wonder if others are experiencing the same challenges and triumphs. Fortunately, online support groups offer a space where you can connect with others who are on similar journeys. These groups can be lifelines, providing encouragement, advice, and the latest information on OA-friendly diets and lifestyles.

Several online platforms cater to people managing OA through diet and lifestyle modifications. Facebook, for example, hosts numerous groups where people share their personal experiences and practical advice on incorporating anti-inflammatory foods, choosing supplements, and staying motivated. These groups are often private, ensuring a space where members can speak freely and seek advice without outside judgment.

Another valuable platform is Reddit, which offers subreddits like r/Osteoarthritis, where individuals share tips, ask questions, and post updates about their diet and pain management. The beauty of Reddit lies in its anonymity, allowing people to discuss sensitive topics without revealing their identity. This anonymity can encourage more candid discussions and allow for genuine community support.

For those who prefer structured discussions, online forums dedicated to health topics, such as HealthUnlocked and MyArthritis, provide moderated environments where medical experts occasionally weigh in. These forums are stored in searchable databases, allowing users to comb through past discussions and find advice on specific OA-related dietary concerns. Being able to search through years of posts means that even if you're shy about asking questions, you can still find answers.

The collective wisdom in these communities is immense. People share what foods have worked for them, discuss recipes, and sometimes even coordinate virtual potlucks where they can all try out new anti-inflammatory recipes together. Users often exchange practical tips, such as how to find omega-3-rich snacks on a budget or creatively incorporate more turmeric into daily meals.

For those interested in more intimate and directed interaction, some support groups offer virtual meet-ups or workshops. These may focus on specific topics like managing OA pain through diet changes or identifying budget-friendly supplements that actually make a difference in joint health. These sessions can be empowering, as they're usually led by experienced members or health professionals.

Of course, with the vast amount of information available, it's essential to approach these groups with a discerning attitude. Since anyone can join these social platforms, the quality and accuracy of advice can vary. It's always wise to cross-reference any recommendations with reputable sources or consult a healthcare professional, especially when trying new supplements or major dietary changes (Smith, 2020).

One recent study examined the influence of online communities on making lifestyle choices among adults with chronic conditions, such as OA. It found that community members often become more engaged with their health outcomes and are more likely to adopt sustained lifestyle changes after participating in these virtual groups (Johnson et al., 2022). This suggests that the encouragement and accountability these online groups provide are beneficial for long-term dietary adherence.

While participating in these groups, don't be afraid to contribute your own experiences. Successes and setbacks alike can serve to inspire and educate others. Remember, these communities thrive on shared knowledge and mutual support. Whether you are asking questions or offering advice, your input has the potential to help someone else on a similar path.

Overall, online support groups can play a pivotal role in your journey toward managing OA through diet and lifestyle changes. They offer a sense of community and understanding that might not always be accessible in face-to-face interactions. So, don't hesitate to explore these digital spaces; they could be just what you need to help mitigate joint pain and inflammation through dietary changes, while connecting with a supportive network that acknowledges and understands your struggles.

From the Author

As we come to the conclusion of this book, I want to express my heartfelt gratitude to those who have embarked on this journey of discovery and better health. Writing this guide has been not only an academic pursuit but also a personal mission to offer support and practical solutions to anyone dealing with the daily challenges of osteoarthritis (OA) and joint pain. Your interest in exploring natural and dietary solutions as a means of relief is a testament to your commitment to health and well-being.

Throughout the chapters, we've delved into the intricacies of how diet affects inflammation and joint health. From understanding the science behind OA to exploring anti-inflammatory foods and supplements, my aim has been to provide you with clear and manageable strategies. I'm hopeful that these insights have helped demystify the complexities of managing joint pain, offering actionable steps to bring about meaningful change in your life. I believe in the power of knowledge to transform lives, and it's this belief that motivated me to compile this book.

Crafting a guide that's both informative and practical was crucial. I wanted to ensure that the information shared was not just another collection of abstract ideas but a set of tools you can actively apply to your daily life. By offering easy snacks, hydration tips, and practical restaurant choices, the goal has been to make dietary adjustments not a burden, but a feasible part of your lifestyle. The strategies outlined in these pages are meant to be sustainable, encouraging small changes that make a significant difference over time.

I'm inspired by the real-life success stories shared in the book. They highlight the resilience and determination of individuals like you who have taken control of their health. These stories serve as a reminder that each small step, no matter how simple, contributes to a broader journey towards improved joint health and overall quality of life. Your journey with this book doesn't end here; it represents a foundation upon which you can continue to build healthier habits.

If you've found value in this book, I kindly ask you to consider leaving a review. Reviews are incredibly important for authors like me; they offer feedback, provide encouragement, and help guide future work. More importantly, they play a critical role in getting this book into the hands of others who may be seeking similar relief. A positive review can significantly impact book rankings on various platforms, ensuring that more people can discover these potential pathways to relief from OA and joint pain.

Sharing your experiences and thoughts not only aids in the book's visibility but fosters a community of shared learning and support. It's about reaching out to others who are facing similar challenges and offering them the chance to discover solutions that might improve their quality of life just as it has for you. Your voice in this process is invaluable and greatly appreciated.

Thank you for trusting this guide as part of your journey toward managing joint health. I hope the knowledge and insights gained empower you to continue seeking and implementing strategies that suit your lifestyle and needs. Together, through shared stories and collective insights, we can create a supportive community dedicated to health and longevity.

References

- (Anderson, J. W., Baird, P., & Davis Jr, R. H., 2009). Whole-grain foods and heart disease risk. Journal of Nutrition.
- (Arthritis Foundation, 2023)
- (Bode, A. M., & Dong, Z. (2011). The amazing and mighty ginger. Herbal medicine: Biomolecular and clinical aspects. 2nd edition.)
- (Calder et al., 2009) Calder, P. C., Ahluwalia, N., Brouns, F., Buetler, T., Clement, K., Cunningham, K., ... & Trichopoulou, A. (2009). Dietary factors and low-grade inflammation in relation to overweight and obesity. British Journal of Nutrition, 101(S2), S69-S78.
- (Calder, 2010) Calder, P. C. (2010). Omega-3 polyunsaturated fatty acids and inflammatory processes: Nutrition or pharmacology? British Journal of Clinical Pharmacology, 75(3), 645-662.
- (Calder, 2013) Calder, P. C. (2013). Omega-3 polyunsaturated fatty acids and inflammatory processes: nutrition or pharmacology? British Journal of Clinical Pharmacology, 75(3), 645-662.
- (Calder, 2015) Calder, P. C. (2015). Omega-3 polyunsaturated fatty acids and inflammatory processes: Nutrition or pharmacology? British Journal of Clinical Pharmacology, 75(3), 645-662.

- (Calder, P. C. (2013). Omega-3 polyunsaturated fatty acids and inflammatory processes: Nutrition or pharmacology? British Journal of Clinical Pharmacology, 75(3), 645-662.)

- (Calder, P. C., 2015). Omega-3 fatty acids and inflammatory processes. Nutrients, 7(6), 4639-4679.

- (Calder, P. C., 2017). Omega-3 fatty acids and inflammatory processes: from molecules to man. Biochemical Society Transactions.

- (Campbell-Falck, D., Thomas, T., Falck, T. M., Tutuo, N., & Clem, K. (2000). The intravenous use of coconut water. The American Journal of Emergency Medicine, 18(1), 108-111.)

- (Cecil, B., & Walton, H. R. 2016). Sulforaphane in cruciferous vegetables as a joint protective agent. Scientific Reports.

- (Chandran, B., & Goel, A. (2012). A randomized, pilot study to assess the efficacy and safety of curcumin in patients with active rheumatoid arthritis. Phytotherapy Research, 26(11), 1719-1725.)

- (Dai et al., 2016) Dai, J., Jones, D. P., Goldberg, J., Ziegler, T. R., Bostick, R. M., Wilson, P. W. F., ... & Vaccarino, V. (2016). Association between adherence to the Mediterranean diet and oxidative stress. American Journal of Clinical Nutrition, 104(6), 1587-1593.

- (Estruch et al., 2018); Estruch, R., Ros, E., Salas-Salvado, J., Covas, M.-I., Corella, D., Aros, F., ... & PREDIMED Study Investigators. (2018). Primary prevention of cardiovascular disease with a Mediterranean diet supplemented with extra-virgin olive oil or nuts. The New England Journal of Medicine, 378(25), e34.

- (Fan, J., & Giovannucci, E., 2012). Basic principles of dietary prevention of chronic diseases. Gastroenterology Clinics of North America, 41(4), 793-835.

- (Feskanich et al., 2003); Feskanich, D., Willett, W. C., Stampfer, M. J., & Colditz, G. A. (2003). Milk, dietary calcium, and bone fractures in women: a 12-year prospective study. American Journal of Public Health, 87(6), 992-997.

- (Fitzgerald et al., 2018)

- (Galland, L. (2010). Diet and inflammation. Nutrition in Clinical Practice, 25(6), 634-640.)

- (Guedes, A. C. & Sargent, M. 2017). The role of anthocyanins in reducing inflammation and improving joint health. Journal of Nutritional Science.

- (Hagfors et al., 2003; Bhatt et al., 2009; Calder, 2017)

- (Harvard T.H. Chan School of Public Health, 2021); Harvard T.H. Chan School of Public Health. (2021). Whole grains and fiber. Nutrition Source.

- (Holick, 2007) Holick, M. F. (2007). Vitamin D deficiency. New England Journal of Medicine, 357(3), 266-281.

- (Hu et al., 2011) Hu, T., Mills, K. T., Yao, L., Demanelis, K., Eloustaz, M., Yancy, W. S., ... & He, J. (2012). Effects of low-carbohydrate diets versus low-fat diets on metabolic risk factors: a meta-analysis of randomized controlled clinical trials. American Journal of Epidemiology, 176(suppl_7), S44-S54.

- (Johnson, A., Nguyen, L., & Patel, S., 2022). The Role of Online Communities in Chronic Disease Management. Journal of Digital Health, 15(3), 456-470.

- (Jones et al., 2020), (Smith & Brown, 2019), (Lee, 2018)

- (Joseph et al., 2014) Joseph, S. V., Edirisinghe, I., Burton-Freeman, B. M. (2014). Berries: anti-inflammatory effects in humans. Journal of Agricultural and Food Chemistry, 62(18), 3886-3895.

- (Jurenka, 2009); Jurenka, J. S. (2009). Anti-inflammatory properties of curcumin, a major constituent of Curcuma longa: A review of preclinical and clinical research. Alternative Medicine Review, 14(2), 141-153.

- (Ledingham & Doherty, 1992)

- (Liu, S., 2013). Whole-grain foods, dietary fiber, and type 2 diabetes: Searching for a kernel of truth. Clinical Gastroenterology and Hepatology, 11(9), 882-884.)

- (Lowe, A. M. 2018). Vitamin C and its significance in cartilage health. Nutrition Reviews.

- (Marlovits et al., 2004)

- (McAlindon et al., 2013) McAlindon, T. E., LaValley, M. P., Gulin, J. P., & Felson, D. T. (2013). Glucosamine and chondroitin for treatment of osteoarthritis: A systematic quality assessment and meta-analysis. JAMA, 283(11), 1469-1475.

- (Miller, P. & Jackson, J. 2019). Lycopene's anti-inflammatory role in joint health. Journal of Inflammation Research.

- (Muraki et al., 2011) Muraki, S., Akune, T., Oka, H., En-yo, Y., Yoshida, M., Saika, A., Suzuki, T., Yoshida, H., Ishibashi, H., Ohnishi, I., Nakamura, K., & Kawaguchi, H. (2011). Health-related quality of life in symptomatic, community-dwelling Japanese subjects with low back pain: The Locomotive Syndrome and Health Outcome Study (LOHAS). Osteoarthritis and Cartilage, 24(2), 164-171.

- (Rickman et al., 2007) Rickman, J. C., Barrett, D. M., & Bruhn, C. M. (2007). Nutritional comparison of fresh, frozen and canned fruits and vegetables. Part 1. Vitamins C and B and phenolic compounds. Journal of the Science of Food and Agriculture, 87(6), 930-944.

- (Seeram, 2008); Seeram, N. P. (2008). Berry fruits: compositional elements, biochemical activities, and the impact of their intake on human health, performance, and disease. Journal of Agricultural and Food Chemistry, 56(3), 627-629.

- (Shen, C. L., Yeh, J. K., Cao, J. J., Wang, J. S., & Wagstaff, J. R. (2016). Potential benefits of dietary ginger in human health: CGMP evidence. Journal of Traditional and Complementary Medicine, 6, 168-172.)

- (Simopoulos, 2002) Simopoulos, A. P. (2002). The importance of the ratio of omega-6/omega-3 essential fatty acids. Biomedicine & Pharmacotherapy, 56(8), 365-379.

- (Simopoulos, 2016); Simopoulos, A. P. (2016). Omega-3 fatty acids in inflammation and autoimmune diseases. Journal of the American College of Nutrition, 21(6), 495-505.

- (Simopoulos, 2016)(Cabrera et al., 2017)(Masters et al., 2015)

- (Simopoulos, A. P. (2002). The importance of the ratio of omega-6/omega-3 essential fatty acids. Biomedicine & Pharmacotherapy, 56(8), 365-379.)

- (Smith, J. L., 2020). The Reliability of Health Advice in Online Support Groups: A Review. Journal of Online Health, 12(1), 78-85.

- (Stookey et al., 2008); Stookey, J. D., Constant, F., Gardner, C. D., & Popkin, B. M. (2008). Replacing sweetened calorie drinks and food with water or diet beverages facilitates weight loss. Obesity, 15(2), 3013-3020.

- Ameye, L. G., & Chee, W. S. S. (2006). Osteoarthritis and nutrition. From nutraceuticals to functional foods: A systematic review of the scientific evidence. Arthritis Research & Therapy, 8(4), R127.

- Ayache, M., El-Jawhari, J. J., Ghaemmaghami, A., & Vaughn, S. (2014). The role of natural medicines in osteoarthritis management. Journal of Functional Foods, 10, 16-25.

- Baker, A., Jones, M., & Smith, P. (2020). The Role of Omega-3 Fatty Acids in Inflammation and Management of Osteoarthritis. *Journal of Clinical Nutrition*, 59(4), 305-314.

- Bandura, A. (1991). Social cognitive theory of self-regulation. *Organizational Behavior and Human Decision Processes*, 50(2), 248-287.

- Bernstein, A. M., Sun, Q., Hu, F. B., Stampfer, M. J., Manson, J. E., & Willett, W. C. (2014). Major dietary protein sources and risk of coronary heart disease in women. Circulation, 130(10), 817-825.

- Bleys, J., Navas-Acien, A., & Guallar, E. (2007). Serum selenium levels and all-cause, cancer, and cardiovascular mortality among US adults. Archives of Internal Medicine, 167(3), 307-315.

- Bondonno, N. P., Lewis, J. R., Prince, R. L., & Devine, A. (2019). Fruit and Vegetable Intake and Bone Health in Older Women: A 10-Year Prospective Study. *American Journal of Clinical Nutrition, 109*(1), 115-122.

- Brandt, K. D., Dieppe, P., & Radin, E. L. (2009). Etiopathogenesis of osteoarthritis. Rheumatic Disease Clinics of North America, 34(3), 531-559.

- Brown, A. & Smith, R. (2015). Joint Lubrication and Water: The Key Connection. Journal of Orthopedic Science, 23(3), 78-85.

- Brown, A. W., et al. (2013). Frequency of behavior predictive of success in losing weight and keeping it off. Med Clin (Barc), 140(1), 35–40.

- Calder, P. C. (2013). Omega-3 polyunsaturated fatty acids and inflammatory processes: Nutrition or pharmacology? British Journal of Clinical Pharmacology, 75(3), 645-662.

- Calder, P. C. (2017). Omega-3 fatty acids and inflammatory processes. Nutrition Bulletin, 42(3), 245-254.

- Calder, P. C. (2017). Omega-3 fatty acids and inflammatory processes: From molecules to man. Biochemical Society Transactions, 45(5), 1105-1115.

- Calder, P. C. (2017). Omega-3 fatty acids and inflammatory processes: from molecules to man. Biochemical Society Transactions, 45(5), 1105-1115.

- Calder, P. C. (2017). Omega-3 polyunsaturated fatty acids and inflammatory processes: Nutrition or pharmacology?. British Journal of Clinical Pharmacology, 83(2), 145-157.

- Chaganti, R. K., Parimi, N., Cawthon, P. M., Dam, T.-T. L., Nevitt, M. C., Lane, N. E., & Cummings, S. R. (2010). Association of 25-hydroxyvitamin D with prevalent osteoarthritis of the hip in elderly men: the Osteoporotic Fractures in Men Study. Arthritis & Rheumatism, 62(2), 511-514.

- Challet, M. (2020). Role of vitamin C in collagen stability and its impact on osteoarthritis. Current Opinion in Rheumatology, 32(1), 82-89.

- Chandran, B., & Goel, A. (2012). A randomized, pilot study to assess the efficacy and safety of curcumin in patients with active rheumatoid arthritis. Phytotherapy Research, 26(11), 1719-1725.

- Childs, C. E., Calder, P. C., & Miles, E. A. (2019). Diet and immune function. Nutrients, 11(8), 1933. https://doi.org/10.3390/nu11081933

- Choi, H. K. et al. (2017). Dairy Consumption and Risk of Gout in Men: A Prospective Study. *Arthritis & Rheumatology, 72*(5), 739-746.

- Choi, H. K., Willett, W., Curhan, G. (2015). "Intake of Purine-Rich Foods, Protein, and Dairy Products and Relationship to Serum Levels of Uric Acid: The Third National Health and Nutrition Examination Survey." Arthritis & Rheumatism.

- Christensen, R., Bartels, E. M., Astrup, A., & Bliddal, H. (2008). Effect of avocado-soybean unsaponifiables on joint pain: a meta-analysis. Osteoarthritis and Cartilage, 16(4), 399-408.

- Christensen, R., Bartels, E. M., Astrup, A., & Bliddal, H. (2008). Effect of avocado-soybean unsaponifiables on joint space width in osteoarthritis of the hip: A prospective double-blind placebo controlled trial. Arthritis and Rheumatism, 59(3), 648-657.

- Chrubasik, S., Pittler, M. H., Roufogalis, B. D. (2010). "Zingiberis rhizoma: A comprehensive review on the ginger effect and efficacy profiles." Phytomedicine.

- Felipe, X. D., Daher, N. M., Correa, R. D., Macoritto, M., & Seibel, T. (2008). Avocado-soybean unsaponifiables in the management of osteoarthritis symptoms: A double-blind study. Clinical Rheumatology, 27(1), 25-30.

- Felson, D. T. (2004). Overview of osteoarthritis. In Lawrence RC, Felson DT, Helmick CG, et al., eds. National Arthritis Data Workgroup. Estimates of the Prevalence of Arthritis and Other Rheumatic Conditions in the United States. Arthritis Rheum, 58(1), 26-35.

- Felson, D. T. (2006). Clinical practice. Osteoarthritis of the knee. New England Journal of Medicine, 354(8), 841-848.

- Felson, D. T., Lawrence, R. C., Dieppe, P. A., Hirsch, R., Helmick, C. G., Jordan, J. M., Kington, R. S., Lane, N. E., Nevitt, M. C., Zhang, Y., Sowers, M., McAlindon, T. E., Spector, T. D., Poole, A. R., Yanovski, S. Z., Ateshian, G., Sharma, L., Buckwalter, J. A., Brandt, K. D., ... & Fries, J. F. (2000). Osteoarthritis: New insights. Part 1: The disease and its risk factors. Annals of Internal Medicine, 133(8), 635-646.

- Fentiman, B., Farnworth, E., & Smith, J. (2020). Beverages and Their Impact on Joint Health. Journal of Nutrition and Health, 45(2), 335-342.

- Ford, R. (2019). Antioxidants and Their Effects on Reducing Arthritis Symptoms. *Nutrition & Health Review*, 45(3), 215-223.

- Fritschi, J., Hu, F. B., & Willett, W. C. (2018). Dietary patterns and the risk of hyperglycemia, hypertension, and obesity in middle-aged Spanish men and women. International Journal of Food Sciences and Nutrition, 69(6), 693-700.

- Gabay, C., & Kushner, I. (2017). Acute-phase proteins and other systemic responses to inflammation. The New England Journal of Medicine, 340(6), 448-454.

- Goldberg, R. J., & Katz, J. (2007). A meta-analysis of the analgesic effects of omega-3 polyunsaturated fatty acid

- supplementation for inflammatory joint pain. Pain, 129(3), 210-223.

- Grosso, G., Godos, J., Galvano, F., Giovannucci, E. L., Giovannini, S., Kales, S. N., & Berry, M. J. (2017). "Dietary polyphenols and prostate cancer risk: A quantitative review with meta-analysis." Annals of Oncology.

- Gupta, S. C., Patchva, S., & Aggarwal, B. B. (2013). Therapeutic roles of curcumin: lessons learned from clinical trials. The AAPS Journal, 15(1), 195-218.

- Gupta, S. C., Sung, B., Kim, J. H., Prasad, S., Li, S., & Aggarwal, B. B. (2013). Multitargeting by curcumin as revealed by molecular interaction studies. Natural Product Reports, 30(4), 558-583.

- Haaz, S., Fontaine, K. R., Cutter, G., Limdi, N., Perumean-Chaney, S., & Allison, D. B. (2011). Effect of oral vitamin D3 supplementation on peripheral insulin sensitivity in humans: an ancillary analysis of a randomized control trial of vitamin D3 supplementation. American Journal of Clinical Nutrition, 94(6), 1456-1462. https://doi.org/10.3945/ajcn.111.013268

- Harvard Health Publishing. (2020). The anti-inflammatory diet: Is it for you? Harvard Health Blog. https://www.health.harvard.edu/staying-healthy/the-anti-inflammatory-diet-is-it-for-you

- Harvard Health Publishing. (2021). Choosing Healthy Protein. Retrieved from Harvard Health Publishing

- Henrotin, Y., Lambert, C., Couchourel, D., et al. (2014). Dietary modulation of inflammation-induced osteoarthritis. *Journal of Nutrition & Metabolism, 2014*. https://doi.org/10.1155/2014/436503

- Henrotin, Y., Mobasheri, A., & Marty, M. (2011). Is there any scientific evidence for the use of glucosamine in the management of human osteoarthritis? Osteoarthritis and Cartilage, 19(11), 1437-1449.

- Hewlings, S. J., & Kalman, D. S. (2017). Curcumin: A review of its' effects on human health. Foods, 6(10), 92.

- Hochberg, M. C., Altman, R. D., Brandt, K. D., Clark, B. M., Dieppe, P. A., Griffin, M. R., ... & Moskowitz, R. W. (1995). Guidelines for the medical management of osteoarthritis. Part I. Osteoarthritis of the hip. Arthritis & Rheumatism: Official Journal of the American College of Rheumatology, 38(11), 1535-1539.

- Hunter, D. J., & Bierma-Zeinstra, S. (2019). Osteoarthritis. *The Lancet, 393*(10182), 1745-1759.

- Hunter, D. J., & Bierma-Zeinstra, S. (2019). Osteoarthritis. The Lancet, 393(10182), 1745-1759.

- Hunter, D. J., & Bierma-Zeinstra, S. (2019). Osteoarthritis. The Lancet, 393(10182), 1745-1759.

- Hurtig, M. B., Choi, B., & Wilson, J. (2009). Effects of unsaponifiables from avocado and soybean oils on cartilage repair and popular culture investigation. Experimental and Therapeutic Medicine, 77(2), 191-200.

- James, M. J., Proudman, S. M., & Cleland, L. G. (2019). Dietary n-3 fats as adjunctive therapy in a therapeutic setting: Relevance to rheumatoid arthritis. British Journal of Nutrition, 107(S6), S227-S232.

- Johnson, L., & Lee, A. (2022). The influence of diet on osteoarthritis. Clinical Nutrition Journal, 25(4), 345-357.

- Johnson, L., Wei, W., & Thompson, Y. (2012). The Importance of Hydration in Joint Health. Nutrition & Osteohealth, 14(2), 189-194.

- Jordan, J. M., Luta, G., & Renner, J. B. (2003). Serum levels of cartilage oligomeric matrix protein and the incidence of functional arthritis. Arthritis and Rheumatism, 48(1), 168-175.

- Key, T. J., Schatzkin, A., Willett, W. C., Allen, N. E., Spencer, E. A., & Travis, R. C. (2004). Diet, nutrition and the prevention of cancer. Public Health Nutrition, 7(1A), 187-200.

- Kidd, P. M. (2011). Omega-3 DHA and EPA for cognition, behavior, and mood: Clinical findings and structural-functional synergies with cell membrane phospholipids. Alternative medicine review, 16(2), 152-164.

- King, D. E., Mainous III, A. G., & Geesey, M. E. (2005). Turning up the heat: Inflammation is a sequel to endothelial activation in the pathogenesis of hypertension and cardiovascular disease. American Journal of Hypertension, 18(1), 79-85.

- Krasnokutsky, S., Attur, M., Palmer, G., et al. (2010). The Role of Inflammation in the Pathophysiology of Osteoarthritis. *Current Rheumatology Reports, 12*(2), 108–115. https://doi.org/10.1007/s11926-010-0089-z

- Lau, C. S., et al. (2018). Osteoarthritis: Pathogenesis and potential for pharmacologic intervention. Best Practice & Research: Clinical Rheumatology, 15(4), 627-644.

- Lee, Y., Kim, A., & Smith, R. (2021). Anti-inflammatory diet for osteoarthritis relief: A study of omega-3s' effects. Journal of Nutrition and Health, 30(3), 223-230.

- Lippiello, L., Cyr, L., & Hesla, M. A. (2005). The Protective Mechanism of Avocado/Soybean Unsaponifiables on Cartilage Structure. Journal of Clinical Nutrition, 61(3), 247-255.

- Liska, D., Mah, E. F., & McDaniel, A. H. (2018). The role of hydration in health and disease. Nutrients, 10(5), 495.

- Liu, D. (2013). Safety profile of the anti-inflammatory agent curcumin: A human and animal study. BioFactors, 39(5), 635-645.

- Medina, M. W., Krauss, R. M., & Borthwick, F. (2015). A comprehensive view on anti-atherogenic properties of fish oil. Current Atherosclerosis Reports, 17(5), 1-9. https://doi.org/10.1007/s11883-015-0512-7

- Messier, S. P., Glasser, J. L., Ettinger, W. H., Craven, T. E., Miller, M. E., Johnson, C. S., & Burns, R. (2005). Weight loss and exercise for community-dwelling older adults with knee osteoarthritis: a randomized controlled trial. Archives of Internal Medicine, 159(19), 2529-2537.

- Messier, S. P., Mihalko, S. L., Beavers, D. P., Nicklas, B. J., DeVita, P., & Carr, J. J. (2019). Strength training reduces knee pain and improves function in people with knee osteoarthritis: A randomized trial. *Osteoarthritis and Cartilage, 27*(1), 68-77.

- Micallef et al., 2009)

- Nieman, D. C., Henson, D. A., McMahon, M., & Wrieden, W. L. (2010). Omega-3 fatty acids: Role in inflammation and potential applications to anxiety and depression. Advances in Nutrition, 1(1), 45–53.

- Pilz, S., Zittermann, A., Trummer, C., Theiler-Schwetz, V., Lerchbaum, E., Keppel, M. H., & Grübler, M. R. (2018).

Vitamin D and musculoskeletal health. Naturwissenschaften, 12(4), 367-372.

- Prochaska, J. O., & Velicer, W. F. (1997). The transtheoretical model of health behavior change. *American Journal of Health Promotion*, 12(1), 38-48.

- Ros, E., & Hu, F. B. (2013). Consumption of plant seeds and cardiovascular health: Epidemiological and clinical trial evidence. Circulation, 128(5), 553-565.

- Rosell, M., de Faire, U., & Hellenius, M.-L. (2009). Associations between diet and metabolic risk factors in men: the role of carbohydrates. European Journal of Clinical Nutrition, 63(6), 781-785.

- Ruiz-Romero, C., et al. (2010). Proteomic analysis of human osteoarthritic chondrocytes reveals protein disease markers. Arthritis Rheum, 62(3), 899–910.

- Seeram, N. P. (2008). Berry fruits for cancer prevention: current status and future prospects. Journal of Agricultural and Food Chemistry, 56(3), 630-635.

- Shanb, A. A. & Youssef, E. F. (2014). Impact of Adding Water Exercises to Land-based Exercises on Osteoarthritis Knee: A Randomized Controlled Trial. *International Journal of Rheumatic Diseases, 17*(5), 509-515.

- Shoba, G., Joy, D., Joseph, T., Majeed, M., Rajendran, R., & Srinivas, P. S. (1998). Influence of piperine on the pharmacokinetics of curcumin in animals and human volunteers. Planta Medica, 64(4), 353-356.

- Simopoulos, A. P. (2002). Omega-3 fatty acids in inflammation and autoimmune diseases. J Am Coll Nutr, 21(6), 495–505.

- Simopoulos, A. P. (2002). The importance of the ratio of omega-6/omega-3 essential fatty acids. Biomedicine & Pharmacotherapy, 56(8), 365-379.

- Simopoulos, A. P. (2016). "An Increase in the Omega-6/Omega-3 Fatty Acid Ratio Increases the Risk for Obesity." Nutrients.

- Singh, J. A., Noorbaloochi, S., & MacDonald, R. (2019). Chondroitin for osteoarthritis. Cochrane Database of Systematic Reviews, 2019(5).

- Singh, J. A., et al. (2020). Dietary therapies for osteoarthritis management: The role of nutrients and supplementation. Clinics in Geriatric Medicine, 36(3), 369-378.

- Skolnik, N. S., & Ryden, E. (2019). Practical considerations for drug pricing in the prevention of cardiovascular disease. American Journal of Managed Care, 25(5 Suppl), S89-S95.

- Smith, A., & Brown, C. (2019). Fast Food and Healthy Alternatives: The Changing Face of Quick-Service Restaurants. Food Policy Journal, 62(1), 22-31.

- Smith, H. (2020). Tackling osteoarthritis with diet: Helen's journey to joint health. Arthritis Health, 12(1), 45-52.

- Sokolov, A. et al. (2011). Antioxidant role of vitamin C and E in the human body. Journal of Clinical Medicine, 61(4), 215-223.

- Vossen, A. C. R., Buurman, J. E., & Willems, H. M. E. (2021). Relationship between Diet, Nutrition, and Osteoarthritis. International Journal of Rheumatology, 2021.

- Weng, C. J., Yen, G. C., et al. (2012). The in vivo and in vitro anti-inflammatory properties of green tea polyphenols. Molecular Nutrition & Food Research, 56(2), 113-124.

- Williams, J. et al. (2017). Hydration and Joint Function Across the Lifespan. Geriatric Orthopedics Review, 29(1), 23-30.
- Zhang, Y., Jordan, J. M., & Lenschow, A. J. (2018). Risk factors for osteoarthritis: Soluble mediators. *Current Opinion in Rheumatology, 30*(2), 107-112.

Printed in Great Britain
by Amazon